The figures are shocking - around 34,000 people die *unnecessarily* every year in today's NHS hospitals and another 25,000 are *unnecessarily* permanently disabled.*

Amanda Steane's *Who cares?* is just one of these 59,000 horror stories. Her husband Paul went into hospital for minor surgery. After repeated mistakes and neglect by inexperienced doctors and over-worked nurses in dirty wards, Paul emerged a helpless invalid. In constant pain and unable to walk, talk or breathe properly, Paul took his own life.

The NHS tried to avoid any responsibility for what was happening to Paul – letters were 'mislaid', promises were 'forgotten' and key medical records were 'lost'. But a nurse, outraged at how Paul and Amanda were being treated, sent Amanda copies of the 'lost' medical records, and the police started to investigate.

In her own words and through photos of Paul's horrific decline from healthy man to helpless invalid, Amanda tries to warn us about what is happening in many hospitals in today's NHS. She does this, not to place blame, but to ensure that nobody else ever again has to suffer as Paul did.

*Patient safety report – NHS website 2007

"Even though most of us know perfectly well that the NHS is working under an enormous strain and that mistakes are made, few of us would deny that the story told in these pages shows just how dreadful the mistakes can be."

"Every Hospital Manager and Doctor and Nurse in the country should be made to read this painful book."
Claire Rayner

D0550588

Dedication

Who cares? is written to honour the memory of my beloved husband, Paul Steane. Paul, I truly hope you have found peace now that your suffering is over. I would also like to thank my two wonderful sons, Adam and Lee. Boys, I'm so proud of you both. Also thank you Adam and your wife Sam for giving me my first grandchild Connor Paul Steane. Thank you to all my family for the support they gave us during Paul's terrible ordeal. My special thanks go to my mum and late father, my beautiful sister Vanessa and her husband Steve. Then last but not least, I would like to thank every doctor and nurse involved who did really care about what was happening to Paul.

Who cares? is dedicated to all the other patients who are being denied proper care in our hospitals. By writing *Who cares?* I hope that I can help prevent what happened to Paul ever happening to anybody else.

I am also very thankful to Peter for helping me see this book through and extremely grateful to my editor and publisher Neil Glass, my agent Andrew Lownie and our publicist Jennifer Solignac for all they have done to make my diaries, papers, letters and notes into such a powerful story.

Who cares?

One family's shocking story
of 'care' in today's *NHS*

Amanda Steane

Original Book Company

The Original Book Company
Studio 8
8 Palace Court
London W2 4HR

Website: www.originalbookco.com
E-mail originalbookco@yahoo.co.uk
Amanda Steane can be contacted on www.nhs-whocares.com

A CIP catalogue record for this book is available from the British
Library

ISBN-10: 1-872188-07-9
ISBN-13: 978 1-872188-07-2

First text edit by Michelle Looknanan, final edit by Neil Glass

Cover design by four-nine-zero design.
www.fourninezerodesign.co.uk

This book was printed and bound in Great Britain

Contents

Chapter 1

Paul's suicide

For some reason, I couldn't sleep well that night. Paul's breathing was very loud and I woke up just about every hour, drifting in and out of sleep. At around 5.00 am, I decided to get up and do some housework, but then I dozed off again before I could. The next time I looked at the clock it was 6:40 am.

I jumped up off the sofa, scared that I had slept for so long. Had Paul stopped breathing? Is that why I hadn't been woken up? But as I rushed over to him, I could hear his raspy inhalations and exhalations, which reminded me so much of Darth Vader. I took a deep breath myself and felt my panic slowly subside. I went into the kitchen to let Sheba our dog out and then came in a few minutes later to go to the toilet. This time I could hear nothing.

I stood there for a moment, near the door to the bedroom, listening closely. I knew that I was a bit on edge and thought that maybe I was being paranoid, as I had been just a few minutes ago. It was probably all due to lack of sleep. But still I heard nothing. Then I simply thought, "No! No! No!"

I crept closer to the bed and, as I looked at Paul, I saw that around the edges of his ear there was a blue tint, just as there had been the morning before he went into a coma two years earlier. I moved faster now, pushing his wheelchair out of the way to expose the bedside table. On it were two pill packets, which had been full the previous night, but were now empty. One was MST, a heroin derivative that he had been given to help control the pain, and the other was amatriptaline, an anti-depressant. The first would have held twenty six tablets, the second fourteen. That made forty pills

Paul's suicide

in all. Normally he would only take one or two of each a night. I wondered how long it had taken him to swallow all of that.

I opened the top drawer of the bedside table, where I had seen him put the letters he had written the day before. There were two sealed envelopes in there, one for me and one for the boys. I took them out and decided that I would put them away somewhere for the time being. I had a vague feeling that I shouldn't be removing anything from the scene, but I didn't want anyone else to get their hands on these. After all, they belonged to us, our names were on the envelopes.

I looked down at him and his face looked peaceful and relaxed – I hadn't seen it like that for so long. It was an even, creamy colour. He lay in exactly the same position as I had left him the night before, with his left hand up by his nose, which had been itching while we had been talking that previous evening before he went to sleep. His hand still clutched the tissue he had obviously fallen asleep with. He was completely still.

He had told me long ago, and then through me our sons Adam and Lee, of his plans to commit suicide. Recently, in his weakened state, he had constantly reminded me that he could do it at any time now, until sometimes I wished that he would do it just so that I didn't have to hear him talking about it anymore. In fact, he had already tried and failed twice. Finally he had succeeded.

This time I did not wish for him to come back. This time I just wished him well on his journey, wherever he was going. Then the full realisation of what he had done hit me and I felt as though a vacuum had sucked out my insides. Paul was not coming back. I could feel panic rising in my throat and a dreadful emptiness in my stomach. I went into the living room, breathing deeply so I wouldn't faint or be sick. I still wasn't sure what to do. I started to pick up the phone to call the ambulance as I had done so many times before. Then I remembered him specifically telling me not to do that. As confused as I was, I could tell that it was too late for that anyway. I put the phone down and went back into the bedroom instead, just to make sure that Paul really was dead.

Paul's suicide

I did what little I could to compose myself then went into the hall, putting the letters away in my bag before calling upstairs for Adam and Lee to come down. I wasn't sure what I would say to them, but judging from the way they got up out of bed right away and rushed downstairs, they both had a pretty good idea what might have happened. Abby, Lee's girlfriend, had spent the night and she came down as well. As I looked at their sleepy faces and rumpled hair, I thought for the millionth time that they were far too young to be going through something like this.

One of them, I don't remember which one, asked me, "what's wrong?"

"Your father's dead," I said, not knowing any other way to put it, but hoping that my voice came out sounding the way a mother's should at a time like this.

Abby flung her arms around Lee and I reached over and pulled Adam to me. I asked my sons if they wanted to go into the bedroom to be with their father, but they both said "no". They were no more prepared to deal with this than I was. I couldn't get the image of Paul, lying dead on the bed, out of my mind. I could feel his presence in the other room and it was almost like a physical pull. I went over and shut the bedroom door.

After a few moments, I let go of Adam and walked over to the phone to call the police detective who had been investigating our hospital for criminal negligence in their care of Paul. He had given me his mobile phone number some time ago for this purpose. I wondered how many nights he had gone to bed thinking that maybe that would be the night that he would hear from me. I dialled his number and when he answered, I told him what had happened. "Have you called anyone?" he asked me straight away.

"No," I answered shakily, "you're the first."

"You must call 999."

"OK, but are you coming over?" I asked, attempting to keep the tremor in my voice to a minimum.

"Yes," he said. I could tell he was trying to make his voice sound reassuring. "But it will take me forty five minutes to get there. Do you want me to call 999 for you?"

Paul's suicide

"Yes, please," I whispered and I could feel myself trembling. This was real and once we called someone in, they would confirm it and my husband would be dead. I just wanted to get everything over with.

"Sit down now and wait until the ambulance arrives," he told me.

"OK, but hurry."

Adam and Lee stayed close to me, still in their pyjamas. I quickly threw on some clothes, not sure if I would be required to go anywhere once people started to arrive. I thought I might feel less vulnerable once I was dressed. But even with my clothes on I still felt weak.

When the ambulance arrived, I showed them into the bedroom. They had lots of machinery with them, but they could see pretty quickly that it would be of no use. Still, they had to be certain, so they pulled the sheets back and put wires on Paul and turned on the heart monitor. The screen showed a flat line.

One of the men moved Paul onto his back and begun straightening his legs. He had been sleeping in an almost foetal position. I overheard them saying that he had been dead for about four hours. I wanted to shout out "No!" and tell them that he had died at about ten minutes to seven, because I had heard him breathing shortly before that, but I just kept quiet.

A policeman walked into the bedroom then. There was another one in the lounge. Adam or Lee must have let them in. They talked with the ambulance men and then turned to me and told me that I would need to give a statement. I said OK and I'm sure that we must have discussed things further, but I don't remember much of what was said at the time. I have a vague recollection of telling them what had happened earlier that morning, which was pretty much just that I had woken up and then found Paul dead a few minutes later. In the back of my mind must have been the fear that they were looking to blame me and that if I said too much, I might incriminate myself. I was beginning to feel faint by that time.

Paul's suicide

While talking to the policeman in the bedroom, I kept looking over at Paul. He looked so lovely and peaceful. I was terrified at the thought of life without him after over twenty four years of marriage, during which time we had hardly ever been apart. But still I was happy and relieved that the nightmare was over for him. Finally.

Chapter 2

Dying for a glass of water?

Paul Terrence Steane was born on May 6th 1957 in Coventry, the youngest of three children. He had an older brother and sister, John and Carol.

The first time I laid eyes on Paul was at the City Centre Club in Coventry, one of the three popular places to go on a Saturday night. It was the end of May 1975 and I was seventeen years old. He had the most amazing smile and, as I watched him try to chat up a girlfriend of mine, I was secretly pleased to see he was nervous and his chat-up lines not very good. By the end of the night, I had worked my way in there and he had asked if he could walk me home.

We laughed and talked all the way back to my parents' pet shop in Earlesdon, the other side of Coventry to where Paul lived. I found out that he had just turned eighteen three weeks before and had been working as a semi-skilled machinist at Apex Engineering since leaving school at fifteen. We met up again the following night and then every night thereafter. It was a beautiful courtship. We had lots of arguments but more fun and always ended up back together again.

On June 20th 1975, I passed my driving test on the very first attempt. Paul was overjoyed when he rang me up during his dinner hour and we began making plans. I had a little red mini, which I had painted by hand. The idea was that we would collect our friends every weekend and go night-clubbing all over the Midlands.

When we were nineteen, Paul bought me a beautiful solitaire diamond engagement ring from a little jeweller that no

Dying for a glass of water?

longer exists in Coventry town centre. We had our engagement party in November 1976 at the Pilot Public House in Holbrook's. Paul's dad, Douglas, was already very sick, but he managed to attend the party, in a new suit no less. He had lost lots of weight, but he still said he felt like the bee's knees. I never knew exactly what was wrong with Douglas, other than that he had an enlarged heart and kidney stones. Sometimes he would be in a lot of pain and would walk around the room clutching his stomach. He had been in and out of the hospital a few times since I had met Paul, but Paul never let on how serious his illness was. Whenever I asked, he always just told me that his dad had kidney stones.

After a night out, we would sometimes get back to Paul's and Doug would be sitting in his armchair, smoking his cigarette. You could see he was in a lot of pain. Those nights I wouldn't stay. I would just give both men a kiss on the cheek and say good night. Other nights he would be waiting up for us so that we could go and get him a faggot and pea batch (sandwich) or, if they had sold out of that, then pork and stuffing with gravy and crackling from Clay Lane a very good batch bar across the other side of Coventry.

In March 1977, Doug was admitted to the hospital for the last time. Paul's brother, John, was in prison at the time for aggravated robbery, but sensing that Doug did not have much time left, Paul's mum Margaret got special permission for him to be let out to see his father. Although pleased to see his son, Doug's face was so sad that sunny Sunday afternoon as he realised that his son being allowed home, meant that Doug had very little time left to live. There were police everywhere and no one knew what to say to each other.

Douglas finally died on March 16th at 8:55 pm. It's a date I could never forget, as it also happens to be my own father's birthday. As we did every night, we had been to see him. He wasn't conscious and horrible brown fluid was coming out of the corners of his mouth. We all kissed him goodnight and left at around 8:40 pm. Back at Longford, we dropped Paul's mum off at the Saracen's Head public house where she worked and went straight over to a phone box to call the hospital and check up on Doug. It was 9:05 pm and Paul was told that his dad had passed away within the last ten minutes. Paul was devastated. That night I sat up all night with Margaret and Paul, the three of us talking about Douglas and laughing about the funny things he had said and done in his life. We tried not to dwell on the painful last few months of his life. It was hard for me, because he had been ill almost the whole time that I had known him. Doug had been a Longfordian, one of the 'elders' in the village, and he would be missed by many. The town wouldn't seem the same without Doug singing *Whispering Grass* while having a few pints in the Griffin pub, his mate Duffy egging him on with every note.

Soon life resumed for Paul, his mother, his brother and sister. Within two months, Margaret had met another man, Ron. Ron had been divorced many years before and had two children, whom he rarely saw and whom we never even met. He was a nice man, but of course he wasn't Doug and so Paul didn't take to him. As most sons would, Paul didn't see why his mother needed another man, especially so soon after his father had died. How could she? Hadn't she loved his dad? And of course he felt threatened, thinking that maybe he would lose his mother too.

What Paul didn't understand was that Margaret was just trying to move on. She told me one day that when you lose your husband like that after so many years, it makes you realise how short life is and you wonder how much time you have left. Eventually your children will move out and settle down on their own and you will be left all alone. Margaret was only forty six years old when Doug died and still felt she had a lot of life left in her. She was always such a popular lady and people enjoyed being around her. It seemed obvious to me that it wasn't going to be long before she found a companion.

Eventually Paul became so difficult about his mother's relationship that she had to ask him to leave the house. My sister Vanessa offered him a place to live with her and her husband Steve. We waited until Margaret had gone to work one night, then packed up Paul's belongings and left. He had been born in that house and his was a very close family, so it was hard for him. I remember him looking around all the rooms of the house that night as though it might be the last time he saw them.

We began our married life together on April 8th 1978. It was not my day to be a princess with a big church wedding, as I had hoped. But it was beautiful nevertheless and we both loved it. We arranged everything ourselves and had a short civil ceremony in the Coventry registry office. Paul and his mother had recently made up, so she and Ron were able to make it to the ceremony. It was wonderful seeing them together again after having not spoken for a few months. There was no money for a honeymoon. I took the next day off work, but that was all the celebrating we did.

Along with Vanessa and Steve, Paul and I bought my parents' pet shop from them. It was a seven-day-a-week job, as the animals always needed looking after, but we hoped we could make it work. The men kept their jobs while Vanessa and I ran the shop. Unfortunately, it wasn't long before we realised that it wasn't working out and we were forced to sell the business back to our parents.

We had to move back in with Paul's mum and the following year I miscarried my first pregnancy. I was heartbroken, but we began trying again right away. We had managed to rent a lovely house in Bedworth and were busily working to get things ready for our first home when we found out that I was pregnant again. This time everything went well and on October 18th 1980, I gave birth to our first son, Adam. Coincidentally, he shared a birthday with his aunt Vanessa.

By now Paul was working for Talbot Cars as a machinist. He began to notice a pain in his left hand that just wouldn't go away, no matter what exercises and massages he did. He let it go on for about six months before going to see a GP, by which time it had spread to his arm and shoulder. We were scared about the spreading and worried that it might be something like cancer. So we were eager to know the results of the tests carried out at our local hospital. We were relieved that it turned out not to be cancer, but we were right to be worried. Rheumatoid arthritis had been known in Paul's family – his father's sister had been diagnosed with it in her twenties and died from related problems when she was forty two. By now the pains had begun to travel all over Paul's body. He started on the long road of treatment and was put under the care of a specialist consultant rheumatologist.

Over the next few months, Paul became quite ill. He had always been an active person who loved playing football and had won several medals playing table tennis for the county. So it was hard for me to see my once-strong man barely able to walk and on medication all the time. At one point, the bed had to be brought downstairs for a few weeks, because he simply couldn't walk up the stairs anymore. In addition to having to take care of Adam on my own, I now found I had to take care of Paul a lot of the time. But as time went on, we learned how to deal with the disease better and got used to the flare-ups.

Our second son, Lee, was born on February 27th 1982. The rheumatoid arthritis had by now settled into every joint of Paul's body and he had to stop working. After Lee's birth, we decided that the best thing would be for Paul to stay at home with the boys and me to return to work.

In the first few years, we tried what seemed like dozens of medicines. We kept hoping that each new one would be the one to halt the disease, not fully realising that it would never go away and the most that we could hope for was a drug that would slow down its progression or ease some of the pain. I became familiar with medicines I had never even heard of, like the anti-inflammatories feldene, pennacillamine and indocin, or the pain killers coproxamol, paracetamol and codidromol. All of this was in addition to the cortisone that Paul had to have injected directly into his joints when the pain became too severe. He hated having those, but withstood the excruciating pain for a few moments of relief and the chance to walk around for a while and play with his sons.

By 1992, Paul's arthritis had progressed to a stage where he was prescribed steroids (prednisolone). Gradually the pain began to ease. We were particularly grateful, as the arthritis had begun to attack his ribs and chest wall, so it hurt him to breathe. Sometimes the pain was so intense that he would break down in tears. I had to struggle to control mine, knowing that I couldn't do

11

Dying for a glass of water?

anything to help him. Though the steroids made things a bit easier for a while, they brought their own problems with side effects like high blood pressure, which meant taking even more drugs. Still, it was so nice to see him able to move freely again and even get down on the floor to play-fight with Adam and Lee or kick a ball around with them in the park. Both our boys played for local Sunday football league teams. Paul became manager of one of them and took part in training sessions. He was now able to do a lot of things that his arthritis had kept him from doing in the preceding years. Also, he could decorate the house and see to some minor repairs. Perhaps it was because things were finally looking up that what happened next hit us so hard.

Paul began to suffer from minor stomach problems due to the wide variety of medications he was taking. It became a vicious cycle, trying to control one problem caused by medication with a different medicine, which in turn caused its own problems. In 1996 he was diagnosed with steroid induced diabetes caused by the drugs he had been given to treat his arthritis. In addition to diabetes, being on steroids for too long can also result in brittle bones and many other problems, so the doctors were eager to reduce Paul's dosage of steroids and try another drug.

Cyclosporine had been used successfully in kidney transplants and had been found to be effective in controlling rheumatoid arthritis as well, so we were very hopeful that it would work well with Paul. The doctors never completely took him off the drug they were replacing though, which to this day I do not understand. I know that steroid dosage needs to be reduced gradually, to give the body time to begin producing its own, but surely one day it can be cut out completely if the patient is being given something else? And it wasn't just the steroid drugs that they insisted on keeping Paul on. Sometimes I wonder if Paul would still be around today if he hadn't been put on so much medication.

Though Paul had experienced health problems since his arthritis started in his early twenties, the beginning of the end – in my mind anyway – came in May 1999. Paul was admitted to hospital with blood in his stools and very bad diarrhoea. He had

12

Dying for a glass of water?

been ill the whole weekend before and was put into a short-stay ward while he was assessed to see if he had a stomach bleed. They put him on a drip because he was losing a lot of fluid from having such bad diarrhoea and didn't seem to be able to eat or drink anything. Later they decided that they would do a camera test in his stomach on Friday, in four days time. He would remain in the hospital until then and was moved to another ward. But even though he still had diarrhoea, he was taken off the drip.

It was unlike Paul to have no appetite. When he had been in the hospital before, he would have me sneak in little treats for him, since he didn't like the food they served. But he wasn't interested in any of that now. I tried to encourage him, but all the snacks remained untouched on his bedside table. Every day Paul seemed to get a little worse and I noticed that he was twitching and becoming confused and sleepy all the time. I was worried, but assumed that the hospital staff knew what they were doing. That Thursday evening, at around 7.00 pm, I mentioned to a nurse that Paul had not been passing urine. She told me that I was wrong and that he had passed water at 9.00 am. What she wasn't taking into account was that, due to the diabetes caused by the medicine he had been taking for his arthritis, Paul normally passed water quite often. I had also noticed that his mouth and lips were very dry and was told by a doctor to give him glucose tablets. He did manage to take a few of these. But still he wouldn't eat or drink and would fall asleep sitting on the edge of his bed. I would have to catch him and push him back onto his pillows so that he wouldn't fall. His sugar levels dropped to below 2 one evening. They should be between 6-10. The nurses seemed to panic and tried giving him milk and biscuits to get his sugar level up.

The camera test on Friday came back negative for stomach bleeding, but the hospital still wanted to keep him under observation. On Monday they moved him to the rheumatology ward, thinking that his illnesses might be connected to his arthritis medication. Even though the tests for stomach bleeding were negative, I knew there was something wrong with him, I just didn't know what. He had begun itching all over, in addition to the twitching and sleepiness. He simply wasn't himself. I decided on

13

Dying for a glass of water?

the Tuesday that I needed to get a second opinion, by this time Paul had been in hospital for over a week and seemed to be getting worse by the day.

I met with a second doctor the next day, who reassured me that nothing was wrong, as the tests for the stomach bleeding had not found anything. When I told him about the symptoms Paul had, he said that he hadn't noticed any twitching. Moreover, Paul had not fallen asleep in front of him. Still, to ease my mind, he agreed to do a blood test. The results of the blood tests came in about 9.00 that evening, after I had gone home from visiting. They revealed that Paul was in complete kidney failure due to dehydration. Had he continued on as he was, he would have been dead by morning. All of this was caused by one very simple factor – he had been taken off the drip eight days before and since then, he had not been given enough water.

Because he was dehydrated, his creatinines, urea and potassium had risen to a dangerous level. Without fluid to control the salts, his organs would have shut down in the middle of the night due to the chemical imbalance in his body. He would have simply stopped breathing and no one would have noticed until it was too late. How could this have happened under the watchful eyes of a hospital? Not only had they not given him proper fluids, but they had been slowly poisoning him. They had continued giving him his medication three times a day, which should never be taken without food or drink. I was appalled, not only by the negligence of the staff, but also by my failure to notice that my own husband was not getting enough water. It's not something you think about when visiting. I suppose I had just assumed that the doctors and nurses would take care of his basic needs such as the two litres of fluid that an adult needs each day. After all, they were supposed to be the professionals and this was such a basic need.

That night I was awoken very late by the phone ringing at home. It was the hospital, telling me that Paul had taken a turn for the worse. When I got there, I was shocked to see that he was surrounded by doctors and on a heart monitor. One doctor stayed up with Paul all night making sure that the fluid was being pumped in correctly. Due to the seriousness of the situation, he did it by hand. They told me that Paul was in a critical condition and might not make it - the next forty eight hours would be crucial. That night stands out in my mind as one of the worst in my life. Unfortunately it was the first of many such to come. I sat beside Paul's bed the whole night, shocked, stunned and not fully realising what was going on. What I found so disturbing was that, if I had not insisted on his blood tests, he would have just passed away in the night and I would have been told that he had died of kidney failure or heart failure. I would have accepted that, assuming that he just had a bad heart or kidneys, and not questioned whether anything could have been done for him. Meanwhile, the truth was that with a little bit of water, all of this could have been avoided.

Luckily, Paul's heart and will were strong and he pulled through. We were both relieved that the reason for his illness had been identified and he could now be treated properly. But we were appalled at the fact that the trained medical staff had overlooked such a basic need as enough water to drink. Once Paul was back home, we decided to consult a solicitor.

I went to see a lawyer and explained to her everything that had happened to Paul while he was in hospital. She told me that yes, indeed, we did have a case. We had Paul examined by a nephrologist (kidney specialist) in London, who stated in his report that Paul's kidney failure was caused by dehydration due to bad clinical care and lack of food and water. Despite all this, we later learned that we could not expect any compensation as, according to the hospital, there was no 'causation' (lasting damage done to Paul by them).

Paul began seeing a local renal specialist, who told us that his kidneys were not diseased, but being on medication for so many years had impaired their function slightly. He needed to take extra care of them, which meant drinking enough water to ensure that his kidneys were properly flushed out every day. She went on to explain that we all need two litres of fluid a day and that if you have been dehydrated to the stage of kidney failure that Paul had been, after more than eight days in hospital without regular fluid, the next time his kidneys could fail in just five days. From that day, Paul started drinking water regularly.

Unfortunately this was just the start of our troubles. When Paul had been bedridden while critical, the hospital staff had forgotten to give him the stockings needed for combatting blood clots. As a result, Paul ended up with a very large clot in his leg. He was started on warfrin, which thins the blood, and sent home wearing the stockings he should have been given whilst bedridden. We had only been home for a few days when Paul had to be readmitted to hospital, this time because he was finding it very difficult and painful to breathe. It was found that part of the clot had broken off and ended up in his lungs, causing what they called a pulmonary embolism. As awful as this was, once again we were very lucky as normally the blood clot goes to the heart killing the patient quite quickly.

Warfrin is generally taken for six months, but they decided that Paul should be on it a bit longer and some doctors even thought he might need to stay on it for the rest of his life. However, some weeks later, Paul developed a rash on his left leg and none of the doctors could determine what was causing it. Paul's diabetes consultant thought it might be a reaction to the warfrin, so he took Paul off it and had him try another blood-thinning drug called heparin for a while. For the next four weeks, I had to give Paul heparin injections, directly into his stomach. I was used to administering his insulin, but these injections were a lot bigger and it took me a while to get the hang of it.

When the rash didn't clear up, the heparin was stopped and Paul was put back on the warfrin, which he remained on for over a year. At that point, during a routine diabetes appointment, the doctor on duty decided that he had been on it long enough and he should stop taking it. Paul and I were both worried, as we remembered that several of the doctors thought that Paul might have to be on it for life. We wondered if this doctor had even read Paul's file. Did he know that Paul had had a blood clot which had led to a pulmonary embolism and that was why he had been put on warfrin? Shouldn't these sorts of drugs be reduced gradually, rather then stopped all of a sudden? One of Paul's worst

16

nightmares was of having another blood clot and of this leading to a stroke. So we decided to get a second opinion before stopping the drug. The next day Paul had an appointment with his renal consultant, so we asked her what she thought. She recommended cutting down on the warfrin gradually over a two-week period, so that's what we did.

Three weeks later, after stopping the warfrin, Paul began to complain of pain in his left foot. We had an appointment to see his rheumatology consultant that week. He took a look at Paul's foot and noticed right away that several of his toes were going blue, the little toe being the worst. It was off to casualty once again. At first they thought that the blood supply was not getting through to his toes, but after doing an ultrasound scan they ruled out this possibility. Since they hadn't yet been able to determine what was wrong with Paul's foot, they admitted him to the hospital to be assessed. There the pain worsened, so they began to administer MST to control it. This was our introduction to the drug and as I did with everything that Paul took, I looked it up to find out more. I learned that it was a morphine-based drug, a heroin derivative.

By the next day, several of the doctors thought that the little toe might have to be amputated, as it had gone very black. They held off though to see if there might be any improvement. One of the doctors thought that it might be another blood clot. If that were the case, then coming off the warfrin was probably what had caused it. Fortunately it had gone to his toes this time. Once again, we were amazed at the thought that all of this stemmed from not getting enough water the last time he had been in hospital. But we tried to remain positive and consider ourselves lucky that it was not more serious.

When I went to see him on Friday, Paul seemed a little worse, but I put this down to the MST that he was taking. He was very sleepy and confused and would often talk nonsense, then drop off to sleep in the middle of it. Paul was so out of it, that he was unable to keep track of how much water he was drinking and I was confused as the symptoms of MST are quite similar to those of renal failure. I assumed that since I had warned the staff several

Dying for a glass of water?

times of Paul's water requirement, they would be monitoring his water intake and urine output. After all, shouldn't a patient who was on a drug as strong as MST be monitored at all times anyway?

Sunday the 18th was Father's Day and, as it was a lovely day, I thought I would take Paul outside for some fresh air. I started to get him ready and put him into a wheelchair while waiting for Adam and Lee to come and join us. As I was moving Paul, he began talking about things that had happened years ago as though they had only just happened. I started to get scared. I ran back to the ward and asked to see a doctor, but my request wasn't received very well. The staff seemed to think that I was just trying to cause trouble and the sister on duty looked at me as though I was challenging her and questioning her authority. The truth is I was just frightened and scared. After our previous experience, I didn't want to take any more chances.

While we were waiting for the doctor, one of the other patients told me that Paul had not seemed very well that morning. When he woke up he couldn't understand why he was in hospital. The gentleman said that he had informed the sister on duty that Paul seemed overly confused and that she had told him to take no notice of it. The sister told him that Paul was always pulling people's legs and larking about. I'm not sure what made her think she knew anything of the sort about Paul, but anyway that had been around 8.00 am and it was now 4.00 pm.

Finally a doctor came and I told her my fears that Paul might be going into renal failure again. When I described his previous symptoms, she agreed that this might be the case and ordered blood tests. I couldn't understand why none of the staff had noticed the signs that were so obvious to me and I had no medical training at all! Why hadn't he been put on a fluid chart when I had told them so many times that he had to drink at least two litres a day?

The tests came back that evening and confirmed that Paul was going into renal failure again. I was furious. The sister I had spoken to before came in with a fluid drip that was, by now, urgently needed and just moved me out of the way with her body, not even bothering to speak to me. I knew she was annoyed with me, but what had she expected me to do? Sit there and let my husband die and not make a fuss? What would she have done if it was one of her family members in his place? It finally made me realise that Paul would never be safe in hospital without his family to look after him. Normally Paul himself would be responsible for ensuring he drank enough water. But how could anyone be expected to monitor how much water they are drinking when they are heavily medicated on morphine? I began to wonder whether there weren't other people in a similar situation, particularly the elderly and disabled. At least Paul had me to keep an eye on things. What about those people who had no one to make sure that they received the proper care?

Once the intravenous fluid was introduced, Paul began to recover quite quickly. I had called Paul's consultant nephrologist and asked her to pay us a visit to make sure Paul was OK. She came the following day at around 2.00 pm. When she found out what had happened, she was rightly angry with the staff and frustrated about the whole situation. She asked for his medical files and wrote in very large letters in red ink, "This patient suffers with renal impairment," in the hope that there would be no more mistakes.

Paul was allowed to go home by the end of the week, although they still were not sure what had caused the problems with the toe. A clot was the most likely possibility and we were told that if the little toe did not fall off on its own during the next few months, then they would amputate it. The other toes returned to normal. We weren't exactly pleased, but then considering that the clot could have gone to his heart or his lungs, the loss of his little toe didn't seem so bad.

Chapter 3

It happens a third time

We returned home and Paul's pain worsened. He continued taking the MST and I made sure he got plenty of fluids. Now that the worst seemed to be over, I began to think about what had happened and how to prevent it in the future. How could I make sure that my husband would be properly cared for if I was not there to see to it myself? It really worried me that both times he went into renal failure, it was I who had notified the hospital staff of his condition. Weren't they supposed to be the professionals? So I wrote a letter to the chief executive of the hospital. In the letter, I explained what had happened to Paul. I tried very hard to come across as concerned, but not complaining. I told of the way the sisters and nurses had treated me after I had brought Paul's renal failure to their attention, which I didn't think was fair at all. I had only been doing what was best for my husband, but they seemed to take it as a professional slight. Paul thought I was overreacting, but I was determined that he would have some kind of safety net in the future.

Again, I thought about what might happen to those who were unable to take care of themselves and had no one to look after them, particularly the elderly. By now I had done some research into the effects of dehydration and knew that the elderly are often affected. They don't drink enough and then major organs start to fail because of the chemical imbalance and, before anyone notices, they die. No one thinks anything of it, because they were old and ill to begin with, so everyone just assumes it must have been their time.

It happens a third time

On the wards, it's usually the hostesses that deliver the water, so the medical staff don't even know how much is being given. The hostesses refill the jugs in the morning, but don't generally monitor how much has been poured out, much less drunk. Many elderly people don't even have the strength to pour themselves a glass of water, not to mention that if you are heavily medicated, you aren't even aware of what you should be doing. Some of the elderly patients have fluid charts when they are admitted, but often the nurses just ask them how much they have drunk, rather than watching them do it. It might seem a bit overprotective to have the nurses see that they take in the proper amount of fluids, but many of these elderly people are simply guessing the amount they have taken in or saying what they think the nurse wants to hear. They don't know themselves the dangers of dehydration and, even if they did, they might not be able to monitor such things themselves. I've even seen nurses just use their own judgement and estimate how much the patient has had to drink, so that it adds up to an acceptable amount by the end of their shift. In this day and age, in a First World country like Britain, it seems ridiculous to me that a lack of water should be a problem for so many people in hospitals.

I sent the letter off to the chief executive at the end of July and a month later I had still not heard anything. By then the toe had become infected and it was more painful than ever. Paul was booked in for surgery, as the toe now had gangrene. There was a three week wait for emergency operations, but at least we knew it would be taken care of soon. At that point, the pain had become so bad that often Paul couldn't sleep at night. He couldn't stand on it either, so whenever we went out, he would be in a wheelchair. Knowing that Paul was going into the hospital again, I began to panic. This time I phoned and asked to speak to the chief executive. I explained to his secretary that I had not received a response to my letter and that I was very worried about my husband. I tried to make her see that it was a very simple case: if Paul had his two litres of water a day, he would be fine. If not, he would die.

It happens a third time

Unfortunately, I did not get to speak to the chief executive, but I did get a call from the regional manager for medicine at the hospital. She said that they had never received the letter that I sent, but I decided not to make a fuss about this and said we could just settle matters over the phone as I didn't want to bother writing another long letter. It might sound ridiculous now, but I actually told her that I did not want to get a phone call in the middle of the night and hear something like, "we're sorry Mrs. Steane, but we lost your husband because we didn't give him enough water."

She said that they would look into my case and what care Paul would need before coming in again and that she would get back to me. She warned me that it would take a while, as they would have to speak to all the doctors concerned. I said that was fine. When she did get back to me, she offered me the option of having their response in writing. I wasn't sure why we needed to have that, but Paul thought we should and she agreed. I requested that if he were in a position where he was unable to look after himself, he be put on a fluid balance chart and have blood tests done every other day to see what was happening with his kidneys. She thought that sounded reasonable and said that they would write to me.

The date for Paul's amputation was set for the 25th September – my birthday. He was to be admitted the day before, but first there was the pre-admission appointment on the 19th September. In addition to having blood tests done and his blood pressure taken, we met with the anaesthetist, who explained that we had the choice of a local or an epidural. Paul opted for the epidural. Next we met with one of the junior doctors, who explained the operation to us and went over Paul's history. She seemed to be paying close attention and writing everything down, so I went away feeling confident.

Paul was to be admitted on a Sunday. But three days before, I still had not received the letter that I was promised. I phoned the regional manager for medicine again. She assured me that it was on its way. She also said that she would come down to the ward to meet with us and put a face to the phone calls. Sunday

It happens a third time

arrived and I took Paul into the ward at about 2.00 pm. He was still on the MST, but a reduced dosage, so he was aware of what was going on around him. He settled in and seemed happy enough, so I left him at around 8.00 pm. As I kissed him goodbye, he gave me a birthday card for the next day.

I rang early the next morning to find out what time he would be operated on and was told about lunchtime. So I kept ringing until it was over and I was told that he was fine. When I went into see him at about 2:30 pm, he seemed well, but in a lot of pain. The toe had been removed and his foot was all bandaged up. We both felt relieved as we thought that maybe now we could finally get on with life and have some fun. He had been in a wheelchair for the past few months, which meant that we couldn't really go out very much. Moreover, we had been afraid to go on holiday in case something happened, but maybe now we would be able to get away for a little bit.

That evening Paul was still in a lot of pain. I asked the nurse if he could have more painkillers, but was told that he had already taken all he was allowed. I asked to speak to a doctor, but when she came around I was told that she couldn't increase the dosage either and there wouldn't be a consultant on duty until later. The doctor said that Paul had already been given 30 mgs of MST. So I explained to her that when he was at home, he was allowed 30 mgs twice a day if he was in pain, so she wouldn't be increasing the dose, as he was already prescribed that. I told her that if she would just look in the file, she would see that I was right. She said that she couldn't as the file was too big. What was I supposed to say to that? A little while later a nurse came around to speak to Paul. Vanessa and Steve were visiting at the time and the nurse asked us if we could all leave while she examined Paul. I was quite upset that she wouldn't let me stay, as I felt a wife has every right to, especially when her husband is on painkillers and not fully aware of what was happening. But I didn't want to make the situation any worse than it already was. I stepped back and she pulled the curtains around them so that I couldn't interrupt.

It happens a third time

I left the hospital that evening with the hope that Paul would have a good night's sleep and wake up in the morning feeling a lot better. The regional manager for medicine still had not been around to see us, but perhaps she had just been busy. I gave Paul a call around 11.00 pm, as I usually did, just to make sure everything was alright. The staff on duty were always quite cold to me when I called late at night or early in the morning, but I no longer cared. My husband was my first priority and I had already seen that if I didn't look out for him, then no one else would.

When I arrived the next afternoon, I found that Paul had been given a higher dosage of MST. He was still in pain and very sleepy, but aware enough to tell me that he hadn't passed water since 2:45 am – over twelve hours before. I told him not to worry, though I was getting alarmed myself and began to look through his charts. There was no fluid balance sheet in there. I got a nervous feeling in my stomach, but I told myself that perhaps they had taken it away to check something on it or fill it out. Paul was sleepy and confused again, but that could have been due to the increased MST. I went to the nurses' station and, after I had stood around for a while, one of them finally looked up and asked me if I needed anything. When I told her that I wanted someone to come and look at Paul, she said she would send someone shortly and that I was to wait at his bedside. I did and no one came. It was getting near the time when I had to leave to pick Lee up from work, so I went back to the nurse. She seemed surprised that no one had been to see me yet and came with me herself at that point. I asked who was monitoring Paul's fluid balance and she said, "no one, why?" My heart dropped. The nurse went out and came back a minute later with an orange book in which they write down the special requirements of the patients. Paul was not in there. I got incredibly angry and explained, for what seemed to be the hundredth time, about his renal impairment and water requirements. And for about the hundredth time, I was told that it would be sorted out.

I told her that Paul hadn't been for a wee since 2:45 that morning and that his water jug was still full. I explained that he was a bit confused from the painkillers and needed to be monitored so that he didn't dehydrate. The sister told me that one of the nurses had said he went to the bathroom at about 8.00 am. I didn't see why they assumed that because he went into the bathroom he had passed water, as he could have been brushing his teeth or doing a number of other things. Why hadn't they simply asked him? Besides which, even if he had been able to urinate then, that was eight hours ago and that's a very long time for someone with diabetes and renal impairment to go without passing water. When I asked Paul a few minutes later, he said that he had gone to the bathroom, but hadn't been able to urinate.

I had the sister's assurances that things would be sorted out now and I assumed that since I had told just about everyone in the hospital about Paul's condition, surely they could not fail to look after him properly. I left to collect Lee and cook dinner for my sons. When I returned at 7.00 that evening, Paul was happy to see me, but said half-jokingly, "what have you done now?" "What do you mean?" I asked. He handed me a fluid chart and a pencil that the nurse had given him. Apparently they expected him to monitor his own fluid intake and urine output, despite the fact that he had just had a toe amputated and was on MST. He couldn't even remember to take a drink, much less write down how much he was having. Not to mention that he was dyslexic and had no idea how to fill in the sheet. Annoyed, I took the sheet over to the nurses' station and explained that my husband was not fit enough to be doing his own fluid chart. The nurse replied that since they were discharging him the next day anyway, a fluid chart wasn't really relevant. I didn't think Paul looked that well, but I was relieved that at least I would be able to take him home the next day and care for him as he deserved to be cared for – like a human being.

Looking back on all of this now, I often break down in tears out of sheer frustration and anger. Why hadn't I just insisted on seeing a doctor when I noticed that there was no fluid chart in his file? Would things be different now if I had acted differently then? Might Paul still be here? But why was it always left up to me to make sure that his basic needs were being met? Surely if you're sick and in hospital, then it is the duty of the hospital staff to look

It happens a third time

after you? Besides, who else could I have spoken to? It seemed as if I had already talked or written letters to all of the doctors, nurses and management. In hindsight, I think part of the reason I continued to believe people who told me that Paul's care would be sorted out was that I couldn't understand how trained medical staff could be so incompetent. How hard is it to make sure that a patient with renal impairment, or even without renal impairment, is given water? Another part of it is that I was just tired of always being made to feel as if I was making a fuss and being an inconvenience. It hadn't got me anywhere in the past, so why should I continue doing it when no one was listening to me? But I was just doing the best I could.

The next day, I arrived at the hospital in the afternoon, happy at the thought that I would be bringing Paul home with me. He didn't look well when I got there, but I assumed that was what you could expect from someone who had just lost a toe. I was told that they wouldn't be able to release him until later that day and, as I had visitors arriving from Plymouth in the evening, I arranged to have Steve pick him up. They got home around seven that evening and Paul looked even worse than he did that afternoon. I thought a good night's sleep was what he needed, so I let him sleep late the next day, which was Thursday. He was still lethargic and confused when I woke him up and I wasn't sure what was causing it, so I decided to stop the MST and see if that would help. He was still in a lot of pain, but there were other painkillers I could give him. I had read that morphine takes about twelve hours to clear out of the system, so I didn't think too much about it when he didn't seem to get better that day.

That night, I finally got to bed around midnight. I was tense and worried, but even with all that we had been through, I never would have predicted what was coming in the next few hours. I don't know exactly what time it was, but probably about an hour later I was woken up by Paul getting out of bed and running to the bathroom. The first thing I thought was 'Paul never runs. He CAN'T run.' But he definitely ran then. I heard a bang, so I got out of bed and went into the bathroom, where Paul was sitting on the dehumidifier. When I asked him what was wrong, all he could tell me was that he was in pain. I helped him out of the bathroom and into a chair in the bedroom, but he couldn't sit still and kept telling me he was in pain. He was sweating profusely and his shirt was already wet through. I tried to get him to tell me more specifically what was wrong, but I couldn't get much sense out of him. I helped him into the living room so that I could keep an eye on him while I phoned the hospital. The sweat was pouring off him by now and when I asked him to tell me where the pain was, he said his lower back and tried to reach it with his hand. I wasn't sure how aware he was, because he didn't really seem to be with me mentally. He looked very confused and his eyes were blank and frightened. I decided to ring 999.

When I explained what was going on, the operator said she would send an ambulance right away. By this time Paul was going in and out of consciousness and I was beginning to get hysterical. Luckily the operator was experienced and spoke to me until the ambulance arrived. She managed to keep me calm and made sure that I kept Paul awake. The relief I felt when the ambulance arrived was physical - finally someone had arrived to help me. I remember thanking them for coming before I began asking questions about Paul. They put him on a heart monitor and said they were going to take him back to hospital. I shouted up to Adam and his girlfriend Nicola that we were taking Paul back to the hospital and not to worry. They were supposed to leave to go on holiday in Tenerife at about six that morning and I didn't want to ruin their plans. I told them to go ahead and just give us a ring when they got there. Then I got into my car and followed the ambulance to the hospital.

Paul was taken straight into coronary care when we reached the hospital and hooked up to an ECG machine. The terminals of the machine kept sliding off because he was sweating so profusely. I had never seen anyone lose so much fluid this way. His t-shirt was so wet that I had to take it off. He was in such great pain that the morphine they were administering wasn't having much effect and he needed my help to move around in an attempt to ease it. I told the doctor that I was worried about the amount of

It happens a third time

fluid he was losing and the possibility that he would dehydrate. The doctor told me that he was waiting for Paul's file to be delivered so he could have a better idea of what he was dealing with. Paul couldn't even stand on his own, so I had to support a lot of his weight and he kept moving back and forth between the bed and the chair. The nurses brought in another chair, an armchair that they thought might be more comfortable, but still he had to keep moving. They tried taping the ECG probes onto Paul at this point, but even that wouldn't hold because of all the sweat. I remember him being so distressed that at one point, when he was sitting on the edge of the bed and the doctor had turned his back to him, he called out, "excuse me, excuse me sir, but can you help me?" It broke my heart to see him that way.

It must have been between 3.00 and 4.00 am when they got Paul's file and I remember the doctor sitting down and reading it. It seemed to take forever for him to get through it, but I thought that at least now Paul would be taken care of. It's funny how people cling to hope. Even though hospital staff had failed me time and time again, I still had faith in their ability to help my husband. So again I expressed my concerns to the doctor and said that I thought Paul should be put on a drip. He told me that he still wasn't sure what was causing the pain and that he wanted to have another doctor come and see Paul first. Then he told me that Paul had been in kidney failure when he was discharged the previous evening. At first the implications of this didn't fully hit me, as I was worried about what was going on right now. But when it did, I was horrified. How could they have discharged him knowing that and not even told me anything about it? Why hadn't the renal team been called now and why was he not on a drip? To this day it amazes me how many junior doctors are put into life-or-death situations which they are clearly not equipped to deal with in our hospitals. Don't we deserve more than that? Don't our loved ones?

The night carried on in this way, with Paul not getting any relief from his pain and numbness setting in to both his legs. I helped him move around as best I could. We were told that a consultant was on the way, but that he had to come from

It happens a third time

Birmingham and wouldn't be there until 7:30 am. Paul was still sweating like crazy and when I asked the junior doctor why, he said it was because of the pain. And still they did not put him on a drip. The consultant arrived a bit after 7:30, perhaps 7:45 or even 8.00. By this time Paul was unaware of anything, but the consultant still addressed his questions to him. He seemed mainly concerned with the problems with Paul's legs and I tried to give as much information as I could, but he kept referring back to Paul. I didn't know if the consultant had been told that Paul was discharged in renal failure, but if he had been, he did nothing about it. No renal expert was brought in and no drip was provided. The consultant went away without really saying very much and did not appear overly concerned. Paul seemed to be getting tired and I thought that finally the morphine was beginning to take effect and maybe he would be able to get some rest. In fact, he wasn't getting ready to sleep, he was getting ready to die.

Foolishly, at the suggestion of the nurse when she saw Paul apparently getting ready to sleep, I nipped home to change and to see to Lee and the dogs. I couldn't have been in the house for more than ten minutes before the phone rang. It was the same nurse from coronary care, who had been with us most of the night, and she said the words I was dreading to hear. "Mrs. Steane, Paul has taken a turn for the worse. Could you come back straight away?"

As I got to the end of our road, I saw my mum and dad pass by in their car. I stopped them to tell them about Paul and, though my mum offered to come back to the hospital with me, I told her I would be OK and drove off. I don't remember much of what I thought on that journey back to the hospital, I just remember being very afraid. I was met by the nurse who earlier had told me to go home. She said that the doctors were with Paul and asked me to wait in a little side room. It's not like me to make a fuss, but I was so angry at her for telling me I could go home that I refused and told her that I wanted to be with my husband. She insisted that I wait and I started to get really nervous. "Is he dead?" I asked, dreading the answer.

"No," she said, "but it's very serious."

It happens a third time

"Why didn't you know it was serious fifteen minutes ago when you told me I could go home? If it's serious, I want to be with my husband," I said, my voice rising and tears coming to my eyes. I was terrified that I would miss Paul's last few moments on earth. I tried to go to him, if only to sit there and hold his hand, but she blocked my way. Finally I backed down and went into the little room to wait. I spent the whole time walking around in circles, with a horrible sick feeling in the pit of my stomach. I expected that any second now a doctor would come in to tell me that Paul was dead.

I'm not sure how long I waited in that room, but it can't have been very long before I couldn't take it any more. I walked back into the ward and this time two nurses blocked my way. I told them that there was no way they were going to stop me this time, so one of them relented and asked me to wait for just a moment while she checked with the doctor. She came back and told me that I could go in. I can still feel the pain I felt then as I ran through the doorway into Paul's room. He was lying completely still on the bed and for some reason the first thing I noticed was that his ears were blue all around the edge. His face was also blue, but somehow peaceful and pain-free. Everything seemed to be going in slow motion. I looked around the room and saw that one of the doctors was holding a bag over Paul's face to keep him breathing. That's when I began to have hope. If she was helping him to breathe, then obviously he was still alive! There were other doctors and nurses running around and seeing to him, but none of them spoke to me. They just smiled sadly. I went to Paul and held his hand, lifeless but still warm. I told him that it would be OK. Then I moved back a bit to give the doctors room to work and sat on a chair willing, begging Paul to live. I didn't know how I would be able to walk down the long corridors once they told me he had died. How I would get into my car and drive home, knowing that the man I had shared my life with for so many years was no longer going to be a part of it. I had never been so lonely in my life. All I wanted was for Paul to wake up and say, "Hi".

It happens a third time

I watched as the doctor in charge made an incision into Paul's neck so that he could put a central line into the main artery. Blood flowed onto the bed, but I didn't even look away because I was just too tired. They were breathing for Paul and setting up drips and injecting drugs. Now they were fighting hard to keep him alive, after having him in the cardiac unit for eight hours, without realising that, for the third time, he was near death due to kidney failure caused by dehydration. They moved Paul into the coronary care ward and within seconds his heart had stopped again. I remember the terrified look on the face of the lady in the next bed, before they had the chance to pull the screen around Paul. Some of the doctors felt that even I shouldn't be seeing what was going on, but I knew that I wouldn't want to die alone and I didn't want my husband to either. More importantly, I wanted to be there if he woke up.

They managed to resuscitate Paul again and then had to arrange a dash up to the ITU (Intensive Therapy Unit) so that they could put him on life support. We all ran through the corridors to a waiting lift and, once in the ITU, Paul's heart gave out once more. They pulled a curtain around him and this time asked me to sit outside it. I listened as they struggled and finally managed to get his heart going again. But that wasn't the last of it. A few moments later they began moving patients around, as they wanted to put Paul into a specific side room. I was told I was not allowed to go into this room, but there was a window so I put my chair beside it and sat looking in. Paul lay there like a piece of meat and doctors and nurses were running around tending to him, trying to get his heart started yet again. One of the nurses saw me looking through the window and came over and drew the curtains. I could still see through a gap though and as I sat there watching, I wondered if she had ever lost a loved one in this way.

I had phoned Vanessa from the coronary unit. She had said she would come over to be with me. I kept thinking, 'God, why is this happening to us? Hadn't I done everything possible to stop it from happening again?' I looked up at the ceiling and thought, 'Paul, if you're up there, get back down here now because you

It happens a third time

can't leave me!' The hospital chaplain saw me and came to keep me company for a while. It was a relief to have someone to talk to, since all the other staff seemed to think I had no right to be there. He offered to go home and get Lee for me, but I preferred to wait and have Vanessa or Steve do it. We talked about Paul and it helped to pass some time and keep me from panicking. Vanessa arrived soon after. I'm not sure if Steve came with her, but he was there later, with Lee and Leanne, Steve and Vanessa's daughter. I felt better having family around me, but could see the shocked looks on Vanessa's and Lee's faces. The ITU is a frightening place and I could tell that neither of them had imagined that Paul would look so bad.

Finally, the doctor came out of Paul's room, along with the ITU anaesthetist. They washed their hands before turning to us and telling us that they had trouble ventilating Paul and so had to knock out two of his front teeth to try to get a tube down his throat. Unfortunately, even this hadn't worked so they would have to try again. But if they were unsuccessful, then they would have to do a tracheotomy (cut open Paul's throat to insert a tube to enable him to breathe). It all sounds so awful when I think about it now, but of course then I said, "yes, do anything you can, please."

He returned about twenty minutes later with a bit of good news – they had managed to ventilate Paul without having to do the tracheotomy. He said that Paul was critically ill, but that we would be able to go in and see him shortly. It seemed like a miracle because all morning long I had just sat there waiting for one of them to come out and say to me, "we're sorry, but there was nothing we could do…" At least now there was a glimmer of hope.

Even with all I had seen, I don't think I was prepared for the sight of Paul when we were let in. The head of the bed was raised slightly and he was on the ventilator, with a pacemaker inserted into his heart and a dialysis machine for his kidneys. In all, there were about thirteen drips going into ports in his arms, neck and groin. But at least he was alive. I went over and gave him a kiss on the cheek and was just so happy that he felt warm.

Chapter 4

Fighting for Paul's life

First thing that morning, I had phoned Paul's sister Carol to tell her that Paul was in cardiac arrest and that things did not look good. I wanted her to be the one to tell Paul's mum in case she got very upset. I assumed she would do it right away, but instead she told me that she was going to see her mum that afternoon about two and would leave it till then. It didn't seem a good idea to me, as Paul might not even make it till then, but I supposed she knew what she was doing and anyway it wasn't exactly the first thing on my mind right then.

Shortly after we were allowed into Paul's room, I was called to the phone. It was Paul's mum, who had apparently rung our house while Lee was still home to ask what Paul wanted for his dinner. He always went to his mum's on Friday for dinner. Lee had told her that Paul had been rushed back to the hospital and was really poorly. Paul's mum sounded so frightened and it bothered me that Carol wasn't there for her. Somehow, maybe because I didn't want to scare her even more, I managed to get control of my own emotions and tell her in a rational way all that had happened. From where I was standing, I could see into Paul's room and everyone was beckoning to me, telling me that he had woken up. I said goodbye to his mum and rushed in to find Paul sitting straight up, his eyes wide with terror. We spoke to him, but he didn't seem to hear us, he just stared into space with a frightened look. A doctor came in and kept saying, "Paul, Paul, it's OK," to soothe him. He did seem to respond and the nurses came in to turn up the sedative so that he would go back to sleep.

Fighting for Paul's life

During the multiple cardiac arrests, Paul had lost about six minutes of oxygen and the doctors weren't sure at what level his brain would function. I remember looking over at Lee and the horrible expression on his face as he watched his once-strong father now reduced to this weakened state, dependant on machines just to breathe. It was hard enough for me, how much worse must it have been for an eighteen year old boy? When we were alone with Paul later, he sat by the side of the bed and held his hand and kept saying to him, "dad, dad, you'll be OK."

A doctor came in later that day and checked all the monitors. Apparently Paul was not responding to the life support. I was told that they expected him to go during the night and that if he did, they would not resuscitate as he was already on maximum life support and there was nothing else they could do for him. The doctor said that they had done everything they could and I knew they had, because I had seen them working on him most of the day. I didn't really understand what was going on, but I knew that Paul was going to die. Lee was with me at the time and became very upset when he heard all this. I knew that I couldn't shield him from what was going on, but I wished that the doctor had taken me aside to tell me about Paul.

Later on, a Spanish doctor who had helped resuscitate Paul, came over to me and asked me if I understood what was going on. I said "no" and she knelt beside me and explained everything. She told me that my husband's condition was critical, but stable. She said that they expected him to have another cardiac arrest because he was not responding to the life support. When he did, if they attempted to revive him, they would have to give him something more to keep him going and he was already on the maximum level of drugs that they could allow. She put her arm around me and told me that if I really wanted them to, they would try to resuscitate him again if his heart failed. I didn't answer and she said that we would just leave it until it happened. Then I could tell her what I wanted. All I could do was thank her.

On the ITU, you have one nurse per patient, so Paul was now monitored at all times, his many drips kept filled and so on. It had been thirty eight hours since I had slept and even then it hadn't been much. It all caught up with me as I sat with Vanessa holding Paul's hand and I felt absolutely exhausted. I was sure this was going to be our last night together and I wanted to make the most of it. I lay my head beside his on the pillow and just looked at him. Despite all the drips and tubes and machines and the assault that his body had been through that day, he somehow looked peaceful. They said that I slept for about an hour, but it seemed to me that I could hear voices throughout.

I don't know exactly what time I awoke, or if I had even been asleep, but in the early hours of the morning it occurred to me that you were supposed to talk to people in a coma. Isn't that what they always did in soap operas and movies? And if you talked to them enough, eventually they would move a little finger or something and then begin to wake up because they love you too much to die and leave you all alone. Of course, I didn't quite expect that, not really, but even if he didn't wake up, maybe Paul would hear me and know that I had been there with him until the end. I didn't really know what to say, so I just said the same things over and over again. "Paul you can't leave me, please don't leave me," and "you won't know where to go without me, you've never been anywhere without me before." I kissed his eyes and nose and cheek and just kept repeating those words. He didn't move his little finger, but after an hour or so the charge nurse came in to tell me to keep on doing whatever it was I had been doing. He said the monitors at the nurses' station showed that Paul was responding. Perhaps it was the rest he had had or perhaps it was me, but at least he was responding. They warned me that it didn't necessarily mean anything and that I shouldn't get my hopes up, but the next few hours passed quite quickly for me as I kept talking to him. And he lived through the night.

As the doctors began to arrive on the ward that morning, they would walk by Paul's room and look in with very pleased expressions. Andrea, a German junior doctor, was walking past our room and stopped and came back in when she realised that Paul was still there. "The one person I never thought to see here alive today was Paul," she said smiling. "Well done."

No one had been able to get in touch with Adam and Nicola yet at their hotel in Tenerife, though Vanessa had been trying and was in touch with Nicola's mum, Michelle. It wasn't until Sunday that Adam phoned home and spoke to Lee, who updated him on what had happened and gave him the number to ring the ITU. I will never forget the pain of that first conversation with Adam. He kept crying and saying, "mum, please don't let him die! Please keep him alive until I get there!" I could hear the heartache in his voice and my thoughts were spinning round and round in my head, but I just couldn't lie to him. I didn't know what to say, so I just held the phone for a few seconds. I didn't know how to deal with this any better than he did, but he was my son and I had to be there for him too. Finally I just said, "Adam, listen to me. If I could promise that to you then I would, but I can't. He is seriously ill and I just want you to come home as soon as possible."

He was crying and he was angry too, because he knew that his father getting sick again had something to do with him being discharged. What he said next struck me straight through the heart, "mum why did you let him go back into that hospital?" He blamed me a bit and I did too. But what could I have done? Let him die at home or try to take him to a hospital further away and let him die on the way? Maybe if I had shouted loud enough at someone, this would not have happened. But there was nothing I could do about that now. In the background I could hear Nicola trying to console him and then she came on the phone. She told me that she would see about getting them back home and I was relieved to have someone reasonable there to look after Adam when I couldn't. He came back on the phone before they hung up and said, "mum, please don't leave Lee at home alone." When I told him that Vanessa and Steve would be taking care of him, he said, "no, he needs you mum." I felt like a failure yet again, because obviously I couldn't leave Paul at a time like this. Not only had I not been able to do anything to save my husband, but I couldn't be there for my sons either. Still, somehow I managed to keep my feelings under control.

What happened over the next few days is largely a blur. Paul's blood pressure was very low, but he continued to respond to the life support and drugs. I don't think he was aware of very much, but then it doesn't seem I was either. Vanessa and Steve seemed to be with me all the time, for which I am very grateful. I don't know how I would have coped without their support. One thing I remember very clearly is the smell of rotting flesh. It's the most horrible smell you can imagine and it got very bad very quickly. Anyone who came into the room would hold their nose. On the second or third day, we noticed a patch of blood on the bed. It was coming from Paul's foot. I suppose that with everything else that was going on, no one had really been thinking that he had just had surgery on his foot a couple of days before.

I had kept in contact with Paul's family, calling his mum and sister on the phone at least six times a day. They also rang the hospital often to find out what was going on, but neither of them had visited yet, which I found quite worrying. By now Paul had been clinging to life for four days. Several other visitors came though, family and friends. The hospital let us use a room just outside the ITU so we could make tea and coffee and just have a break or even a nap in there if need be. I felt lucky to have the friends and family that I did and they said the most beautiful things about Paul, remembering his life and the fun-loving person he had been.

On Sunday the 1st October, after being in the hospital for two days without a break, I was badly in need of a shower. For the first time, I felt that I could leave Paul and he would be there when I got back. In twenty five minutes flat I raced home, showered and raced back. I just had time to give Sheba, our German shepherd, a cuddle. She was excited to see me, but obviously confused by all the commotion of the past few days and about being left alone for so long. Lee and Leanne had taken Belta, our bearded collie puppy, to the kennels, because she was a little too young to be left alone for so long. I spent the rest of that day at Paul's side then left on Monday morning to rush home and shower. On my way out the door I picked up all the mail that had accumulated, thinking I would have time to read it in the hospital while Paul was sleeping.

I sat down to read my mail and in the stack, I found the letter that I had been waiting for from the chief executive of the hospital, concerning the dehydration that Paul had suffered there in the June. It was dated 25th September, the day that Paul had his amputation. I was very cross, as the whole point of my getting in touch with him had been to try to establish safety procedures for Paul *before* his amputation. The letter was three pages long and seemed to be describing in detail how well Paul had been treated when he had first suffered renal failure. I didn't understand much of the letter, but one paragraph surprised me:

Mr. Steane was reviewed later that day by Dr. ------- and in view of his temperature considered whether infection and dehydration were also contributing factors in the deterioration in renal function. Treatment regimes were reviewed, antibiotics and fluids were suggested and the ACE inhibitors were stopped. On this day his renal function was already beginning to improve.

This simply wasn't true. The doctors hadn't noticed that Paul was going into renal failure. It was only because I insisted on them doing a blood test that they found this out. Yet here the hospital management seemed to be claiming that the doctors had been in control of the situation all along.

Also from the hospital was the annual report that went to every home in the area. There was a photograph on the first page of the chief executive. The whole report was so positive and cheerful and here I was looking at my husband, in a coma because he hadn't been properly cared for and given enough water. All that evening I just sat in the chair reading those letters over and over, trying to understand what had gone wrong.

I continued to stay at Paul's bedside for the next few days, becoming heavily involved in his care and treatment. I also learned a lot about the drugs he was taking and which signs were good and which were bad. I wasn't angry, but I needed to know what was going on every step of the way. I also learned how to read all the charts and monitors. It wasn't that I didn't trust the staff, but I just couldn't take any more chances. Here in the ITU, the nurses seemed very professional. They watched over Paul all the time and worked with his body, reducing medications when they thought he could manage, raising them again if it proved to have an adverse effect. Paul was having adrenalin and noradrenalin at quadruple strengths and had been from the start – normally someone on life support would have single or double strengths. That's why they had told me a few days earlier that if his heart failed again, they wouldn't be able to do any more to keep him alive.

I watched as Paul's body fought to live. It was slow going, but wonderful to see. His heart started trying to beat on its own, as if saying "I can do it". The pacemaker might still be doing ninety five percent of the work, but his heart was trying. Then the ventilator started to show signs that Paul was taking breaths on his own, in between the ones that were being taken for him. Small steps, but still steps towards recovery. A couple of days later, one of the senior anaesthetists in charge of the ITU came in. Though I had only known him a short while, I had a lot of respect for him. I had only ever seen him treat his patients and their families in a loving, caring manner. He came in to talk to us and put his hands on Lee's shoulders and mine in a sympathetic, comforting gesture. He said to me, "in all my years of being a doctor, I have never had to come to tell someone off for caring so much." I was surprised at his words, but listened to him without interrupting because I wasn't sure my mind was working clearly at such a stressful time and maybe he had a point to make that I hadn't considered. He told me that one of the nurses had come to him, saying that she was a bit offended at my constant questions and the fact that I stayed at Paul's side all the time. She felt that I didn't trust her and that I was watching every move she made. He said it was hard to find good nurses to stay in the ITU because of all the trauma and stress they faced on a daily basis. He thought it was unprofessional of a nurse to complain about a relative being present, but that just as I needed to have "special moments" with Paul, the nurses did as well. Besides, he said, I should think more about myself and I needed rest too.

I was taken aback by all this, because I hadn't sensed any hostility from the nurses and thought that surely they would understand that I was just concerned about my husband. After all, even though they hadn't been the nurses in question, I had put my trust in hospital staff before and this had led to Paul suffering renal failure three times. Could anyone really blame me if now I was getting involved in everything that was happening to my husband? Besides, why in God's name would the nurses need "special moments" with Paul? I tried to keep my voice level and said that I was sorry if I had offended anyone, but my first and only concern was Paul. If he died, I wanted to be there when he went and if he awoke, I wanted to be the first person that he saw. I think I made it quite clear that I wasn't going to be leaving.

The following morning, I decided to go to the hospital restaurant for breakfast as Paul's condition seemed to be stable. As I was walking along the corridor towards the café, I saw the sister whom I had told that Paul had stopped passing water before he was discharged in renal failure. She was talking to someone and I was undecided whether or not I should approach her and say something about Paul's current condition. I decided against it, not wanting to cause a scene or get myself upset. As I passed by, she turned from the person she was talking to and said, "hello Mrs. Steane. I've heard about Paul, how is he?" I was very polite and updated her on his progress. She said she would come along later and see us. I was proud of myself for being able to handle the conversation in such a mature way, but at the same time I wondered why I didn't shout at her and tell her that I might not have to be here right now if she had only done her job.

I carried on into the restaurant and, as I was at the till waiting to pay, I looked over at the seating area and saw the chief executive at a table, eating his breakfast with three other men all in suits. I checked with the cashier to make sure it was him, as the first time I had seen his picture was the night that I read the report

Fighting for Paul's life

from the hospital. She said that it was the chief executive, but warned me that I couldn't interrupt him and that I should call his secretary and book an appointment if I wanted to see him. I thanked her for her help and, with the conversation with the nurse still fresh in my mind, I put my tray down on a table and walked over to where the chief executive was eating his toast. I put out my hand to shake his and introduced myself. He was very polite as I told him that my husband was in a coma in the ITU and that I needed to see him about it. He said he would speak to his secretary and arrange for a meeting sometime the next week. Next week? I was stunned. I replied quickly, before I lost my nerve, "OK, as long as you can guarantee that Paul will be alive next week. At the moment they are only giving him from hour to hour and I wanted you to see him." He immediately apologised and called his secretary, telling her to look at his diary and arrange a meeting for him in the ITU that day. He then turned to me and said that his secretary would call me in the ITU and let me know what time he would come by that day. I thanked him and went to have my breakfast.

Later that day, a message came through to the ITU saying that the chief executive would be along at 4.00 pm. At about 3:45 two people came onto the ward and introduced themselves to me – the director of nursing for the hospital and the ITU manager. They both came into Paul's room and looked at his charts, telling me that the chief executive would be along shortly. He was, but walked straight into the meeting room at the end of the unit, never coming into Paul's room. Lee and I went along with the two others and the meeting began. They asked me to tell them all that had happened to us and I tried to be as accurate as I could, though reliving all that we had been through was very emotional for me. At the end of the meeting, I thanked them all for listening and we said our goodbyes. No one said that they would look into it or get back to me, I just took it as a given that they would.

Meanwhile, Adam and Nicola still had not been able to make it home. Their holiday company did absolutely nothing to help them. In the end they went and sat in the airport in Tenerife until another company said that they had room on a flight back to England. They had to pay for it, but at least they were coming back. They were scheduled to arrive at Heathrow on Wednesday morning at 3:30 and Adam's best friend Paul Gibson had kindly offered to pick them up and bring them straight to the hospital. So I was expecting them at about 5.00 am.

The nurses knew that Adam would be seeing his father for the first time since he had been brought back into hospital, so they washed Paul early and tried to make him look as good as possible. Normally, the nurses would wash him every morning and night and I was encouraged to help. I would do all his private parts, which was a bit difficult as he was catheterised and I was afraid of dislodging it. I noticed that his breath smelled very bad and, though it seems a small thing, I worried about it because he is such a clean person and he would hate the thought of people kissing him when he smelled like that. It was due to the blood from his pulled teeth and lack of saliva to clean his mouth, as he wasn't breathing and swallowing like a normal person would. I asked one of the nurses if there was anything we could do about this and she told me that I could bring in his electric toothbrush. The next time I went home, I brought it back with me and began cleaning his mouth every day. The smell disappeared quite quickly.

While we were cleaning him that morning, a nurse noticed that the ventilator cords were tied very tightly around his face. Blood had been absorbed into the cords and it was very messy and smelly around his mouth. As she removed the cords to retie them, we saw that they had cut deep into the sides of his mouth and the cuts had become infected. She bathed and cleansed the area and then used fresh cords to put it back in place, this time putting small sponges under them so they wouldn't cut into Paul's skin.

They had advised me to take Adam and Nicola into a side room before they saw Paul, to explain to them everything that had happened and to prepare them for how Paul would look. This seemed like a good idea to me, so when they arrived I went down to meet them. I was so glad to see them walking up the corridor towards me, though they both looked tired and worn. I kissed them and then took them aside to talk to them. Of course they were both eager to see Paul for themselves, so I kept it short and then we all went up to the ITU. When we got there, a nurse came with us into Paul's room. She sat Adam down and explained everything that was happening to his dad, what the machines were doing and what all the drugs were for. Then we left him and Nicola to be alone with Paul for a while.

The following Monday, the surgeon who had originally admitted Paul to amputate his toe, was asked to come back to look at the foot. It smelled foul and there was fluid running from it onto the bed and floor. It was this day that I noticed Paul's other foot – the toes and part of the foot itself had gone black and there were big blood blisters. I was told that this had happened as a result of the noradrenalin. The drug is a vascular constrictor and, though it keeps the blood going to the main organs, it often stops the blood supply from going to the feet. Because Paul had been on quadruple strength since he had gone into a coma, his feet had been severely deprived of blood.

It was around then that I began to notice that every time I left the room, whether it was to go to the bathroom or to get a snack or for any other reason, the nurses would make me wait a while before going back into Paul's room. Unfortunately, I had a couple of arguments with them over it, but they just kept telling me that they needed "special moments" with Paul too. One day, when I went to the bathroom and came back, they wouldn't let me in at all. They said there was a doctor examining him, so I bit my lip and waited. After a while, the doctor came out looking strained. He came over to me and said, "I have looked at Paul's foot and, if he survives this, we are looking at major leg amputation." Once again I was in shock. I hadn't thought there were any more bad things that could happen to Paul. From the doctor's tone, I could tell that he was wondering if Paul's life was worth fighting for, considering what he would have to go through if he did survive. That made me start thinking as well.

Fighting for Paul's life

I went in to have a look at Paul. He was lying so still, looking peaceful and free of pain. Then I lifted the bedclothes and thought, "oh, my God!" His whole left foot was dead, the flesh hanging rotten and black. I had never seen anything like it in my life. I remembered an advert we had seen on TV a few years before. It was part of an anti-smoking campaign and showed a man who had somehow lost his leg from smoking. The advert opened with his little girl crying about her daddy losing his leg. Whenever we saw that, Paul would say to me, "if I ever lose my leg, I wouldn't want to live." I wondered what he would say if we could ask him now. It's true that for many years he had lived with a lot of pain, with his arthritis and all, but he had always been able to get up and move around. He was an independent man, though when he was in bad pain he liked being pampered a bit. Who wouldn't? Sometimes we would have to help him to his feet and when he began to get ill he needed a bit of support, but how would he manage without one leg?

My mind was still in a whirl over learning that my husband might lose a leg, when one of the doctors came in with a nurse and said that they would like to speak to me in a private room. We went down the corridor to the staff room and all sat down. He started off by asking me if I understood how critical Paul's condition was. I said yes, my eyes filling with tears. It was hard to listen to him when I kept seeing in my mind Paul's rotting, black, dead foot. "Paul's heart may not hold out," the doctor said to me, trying to be gentle. "After the assault it has taken, it is very doubtful that he will make it and you must understand that there is still a very long way to go. Even if he does recover, he might have permanent heart problems."

I kept trying to concentrate, but my head was full of questions, the same ones over and over. 'What should I do? What would Paul want me to do? If he survives, what kind of life will he have? Will he blame me for what has happened? God, please tell me what to do!' Later, I sat there staring at Paul's face, hoping he would give me some sign of what he wanted. I looked at the machinery and wondered what I would say if a doctor came to me and said that maybe it was time to turn it off. No one had brought that up yet, but how long before they did? We didn't even know yet how much of his mind was left intact. What if his body came back to life, but not his soul?

By the time the visitors came by that evening, I had made up my mind. There had been signs of improvement and, though they were tiny, they were still there. We would get by, leg or no leg. Paul wouldn't let that keep him down and if he survived this then together we would find reasons to go on.

That same Monday, at around 7.00 pm, Paul's rheumatologist paid us a visit. He was accompanied by a lady I had never seen before and as he sat down he expressed his sympathies and asked me to tell him what had happened. As I began, he interrupted me to introduce this lady – it was the regional manager for medicine who had promised to come and see me. I was shocked, to say the least, but I invited her to sit down and she did. After bringing Paul's rheumatologist up to date, I turned to the lady and asked her why she hadn't come to see us on the ward. She replied that she had, but the curtains had been pulled around Paul and she hadn't wanted to intrude. Then she started to cry. My first thought was, 'God, I really don't need this, especially not today.' But I quickly began to feel sympathy for her, she seemed to be in such pain, so I reached out and put my arm around her.

"This is all my fault, isn't it?" she asked me. Deep down, I was angry with her for not arranging things for Paul as she had promised me she would, but I couldn't let her shoulder all the responsibility. Besides, she did seem to be truly sorry. "No," I said, "lots of people are to blame."

The rheumatologist had been checking Paul over during this time and now he began to gather up his things, telling me he would be back to check on him another day. He held my hand and told me how sorry he was. I thanked him and he left. By now the lady had stopped crying and composed herself. She asked me if it was alright for her to come back and see me the next day, to see how Paul was and if there was anything that I needed. I said of course it was and then she left too. I felt emotionally and physically drained by all that happened that day, but glad that we had made it through.

That Tuesday they decided to reduce Paul's adrenalin as well as his sedative. He had woken up briefly the night before, though not fully, and never opened his eyes. He kept grabbing at the tube and trying to pull it out of his mouth. They woke me up to try to help settle him, which I thought was a bit strange as it was 3.00 am. The nurses had given me a pink reclining chair to sleep on. I tried to soothe him, but nothing I did worked, so in the end they had to turn his sedative up to knock him out. During the day, he began to move about and open his eyes, but he wasn't aware of anything and before you could speak to him, he would fall asleep again. They had coached me on what to do if he woke up, as he wouldn't know where he was or what was wrong and it was important that he remain calm. I was to gently tell him that he had been very poorly, but was now OK. I had to tell him that he had a tube down this throat and, even though it might be uncomfortable, he needed it because it was helping him to breathe.

Paul also had a food line inserted into his nose which went down into his stomach. He had begun absorbing the food, so they increased the amount that they were putting in. That morning I went home to shower as usual and when I came back, there was a horrid smell in the room. It was so bad that I had to put my hand over my face. Paul's stomach had not absorbed the food for some reason, so they had had to empty his stomach, siphoning the contents through a tube into a jug, then piping it back in. For some reason this worked and he absorbed the nutrients the second time around.

The day before, they had begun physiotherapy. Mainly they would do breathing exercises designed to make him cough. As he coughed, they would use suction to bring up the mucus in his lungs and help keep them clean. It was very unpleasant to see, but I suppose it had to be done. They also did some work on his arms and legs, to keep the muscles from atrophying. We noticed that his foot kept shaking and thought he might be in pain. I remembered that when his little toe went bad, it hurt him to have anything touching it, even a sheet. I asked the nurse if they could get a cradle to put on the bed, that way the blankets wouldn't actually be touching his feet. They found one and as I was arranging it, I got a better look at his legs and feet. It was awful – the fluid leaking from them was soaking the bed and the smell was horrendous. When I left the room it went with me, it seemed to be in my clothes and nostrils.

Later that day, as I was tidying Paul's bed, making sure that nothing was touching his feet, I happened to look up and saw him looking back down at me. I ran up to the top of his bed and his eyes followed me. "Hello!" I said, kissing him, so excited, but trying to remain a bit calm so as not to frighten him. "Paul, you have been very ill and have a tube in your mouth to help you breathe. Please don't worry, I know it's not nice, but you need it right now." I had rehearsed what I would say to him in my mind so many times, praying that I would get the chance to actually say the words. He nodded and I felt a flood of relief that finally he was responding to me and that he understood what I was saying. He was wrapped in foil at the time, to keep him warm. I asked him if he was cold and he shook his head 'no'. I was ecstatic, because if he could answer questions, even if he couldn't speak, then his brain was probably not damaged. I looked at him for what seemed like hours and then remembered that I should probably inform the nurses.

I was torn between the desire to stay with my husband, just holding him and telling him I loved him, and going out to tell his sons and the rest of our family that he had woken up. But I knew the boys would want to know as soon as it happened and it wasn't fair to them for me to be selfish, so I ran out to the callbox. I phoned them, both our mums, Vanessa and I can't remember who else, but only very quickly, and then rushed back to be with Paul. He had fallen back asleep by the time I got there, but that was fine. At least now I knew he would be alright. I just sat there and waited for him to wake up again. When he did, I was grateful to see that he looked so happy to be alive. I had been afraid that he might not want to go on. Of course I was aware that he didn't yet know what was in store for him, but at least he had the will to survive. We could get through anything as long as he had that.

As I think back, I'm amazed at how he took everything in his stride. He looked around at all the drips and monitors. Of course he was scared, but not overwhelmed as some people might have been. He found the ventilator difficult to deal with, but understood that he needed it. He tried hard not to show that he was nervous and greeted everyone with a smile. He was so brave and I was so proud of him.

Over the next few days, we talked a lot. Or at least I talked and he communicated to me by nodding or making other gestures. On one occasion he turned his head towards me and mouthed, "I love you," then pointed upwards with his hands and mouthed, "you and I are going up." He meant that we had been given another chance and we would make it. I started to cry and leaned over and kissed him. I loved him so much. I knew that we still had a long way to go, that in a sense the battle was only just beginning, but I knew that we could make it. On some days he took a turn for the worse and one day they had to call a doctor from Birmingham because his veins had collapsed from all he drugs he had been given over the last few days. When she came out to see me, she said, "your husband is still a very ill man and it could still be a tragic outcome." I was aware that just because he was awake and happy now, it didn't mean that he still couldn't die at any moment. But I didn't care about that right now, all I cared about was that Paul was still alive.

Chapter 5

Widespread neglect

Every day Paul would be awake a little bit more and I noticed that he spent quite a bit of time just staring up at the ceiling. He would look around the edges of the room, but his eyes were focusing on something, it wasn't just a blank stare. I asked him what he was looking at, but he didn't know how to communicate it to me. He had a really excited look on his face though and I felt I knew what he wanted to say.

"Have you had an out-of-body experience?" I asked him. He nodded, but gave me a look that said, "don't worry though, I'm not crazy. It's OK. We'll talk about it some other time." I knew him so well that even though he couldn't speak, I could understand what he meant just from glances and gestures. Sometimes he would write little notes to explain what he wanted and those always made me smile because he was dyslexic. He would write all in capitals using only small words, but all joined up. He couldn't put a sentence together properly and you would have to guess what he was trying to say. It was easy for me, but others had quite a difficult time understanding. He himself found it quite funny and I was so glad to see that his sense of humour had not been affected by all that had happened. He could make anyone laugh and that was one of the things I had fallen in love with.

I was worried because he hadn't had a movement since he'd been readmitted, but finally on October 8th he opened his bowels for the first time. I was so relieved that the nurses began laughing at me. Obviously it happened in bed and changing the sheets was a lot of work. Every time we moved him, Paul would scream in pain. It was very unusual for him, because he was used to pain from his arthritis, so we knew it must be very bad. He also had a lot of pain in his chest and the doctors thought that maybe some of his ribs had been broken when they tried to keep him alive manually on the 29th September. It would take four nurses to change the bed: three to roll him over while the other one pulled out the sheet and put a new one on. Often we had to wait a little while before four nurses could be rounded up at the same time and on this particular day it didn't happen until 4.00 pm. By then Paul had done another poo in bed. I was beginning to get worried about him lying in his own waste for so long, so I mentioned it to one of the nurses and she sorted it out. The doctors began to talk then about taking the ventilator out. It had already been in longer than it should have, but they were reluctant to remove it because it had been so difficult to get it in there in the first place. They were worried that if it turned out they had to put it back in, they wouldn't be able to. Finally the decision was made and on Tuesday 10th October at 3:15 pm, they came in to remove it.

I couldn't wait to hear Paul's voice again and of course he was very anxious as well. I found it amazing that only a few short days ago no one knew whether he would live or die. Now he was getting ready to come off the ventilator and start speaking. Paul was very scared that he wouldn't be able to breathe on his own, but I didn't see how any harm could come to him when he was surrounded by doctors.

Paul hadn't slept very well the night before. His left foot had been hurting him a lot. He still hadn't been told what was going on with his feet and leg, all he knew was that he had had a toe amputated. He asked me to show him his foot, so I pulled back the sheet from his foot and held my breath as he had his first look at it. He looked so shocked and was trying to ask me what had happened. I told him not to worry, that things would be alright. I didn't know exactly what to tell him, so I just told him the truth: that the amount of noradrenalin that had been required to save his life had cut off the blood supply to his foot. I had thought that maybe the idea of the ventilator coming out later that day would take some of the sting out of seeing his foot, but how could I expect him not to worry? I can only imagine how awful that first sighting must have been for him, with all the rotting, hanging flesh and the blisters full of blood and fluid. And he hadn't even seen his other leg yet. I didn't think he could take the shock of that right then, so I pulled the covers back up and went to the top of the bed and kissed him gently. I tried to distract him by talking about other things.

A little while later, the physiotherapist came along. She had been looking after Paul while he was in a coma. It's quite important to keep the airways clear so that secretions don't build up and encourage infections. At the time, Paul's secretions were quite thick and it was hard for him to get them up, so he had been having physio twice a day. However, up till then he had been unconscious. Now that he was awake, the experience was quite traumatic for him, but he faced it bravely. The physiotherapist decided to work his legs then and, before I could stop her, she pulled the sheets back revealing both his feet. The right was nowhere near as bad as the left, but it was still damaged and I could see Paul looking at me and questioning with his eyes. The physiotherapist immediately realised and turned to me and asked, "didn't he know?" "No, but it's OK," I said, trying to make light of the situation.

Once she had finished and left us alone, I explained to Paul what had been going on. I told him that yes, it was true that the right foot was also affected, but only the toes and they may still go back to normal. I didn't want to give him any false hopes though, so I told him that there was also a chance that they might not get better at all. The condition of his feet depressed him for a while, but I was glad that I no longer had to hide it from him. After all, he had begun to notice the smell as well, even if he didn't necessarily know where it was coming from. At least now we could start to deal with the issues that we had to face together. During his coma, I had to be strong for both of us, but it was exhausting and now that he was back I needed to be able to rely on his strength too. I wanted to cry with him, but I knew it would be selfish. He was the injured one and I had to let him see that I believed we could make it.

They came on time to remove the ventilator and when the tube came out, it felt as if we had just passed our first milestone on the way to Paul's recovery. "Hello," he said to me and I burst out crying. "I love you Paul, well done," I managed to get out through my tears, kissing him at the same time. God it was good to hear his voice again! We spent the rest of the day talking. After not being used for so long, his voice was a bit husky, but it was still his. I asked him about his staring at the ceiling and he said that somebody was looking after him. He didn't know why, but it didn't scare him at all. He had mentioned having an out-of-body experience and he told me more about that now. He said that it had happened on the 29th September, while he was in the coronary care unit. He said that he remembered looking down at his own body and that he could see me and lots of other people as well. He described them to me and then recounted everything that had gone on while we were in that room. It was completely accurate.

He said that an old man had been with him, but when I asked him if it was his dad, he said "no". He didn't know this man or where he was from or why he was there, but he had stayed with Paul and made him feel safe. It was very peaceful, he said, and he had no thought of living or dying. He had just been observing what was going on and enjoying the beautiful feeling of not having any worries. The man had been with him in the ITU as well, he went on, and would stand directly behind me a lot of the time, just smiling at us. Paul hadn't seen him for a few days, but he wasn't worried about it. He just assumed that maybe he didn't need him anymore now that he was getting better. We both had a good laugh about the whole thing because Paul had never been religious or spiritual and hadn't thought much about life after death. But here he was seeing spirits and now he definitely believed that there was an afterlife. He wouldn't be scared to die when his time came, he said.

Ever since hearing that the ventilator was going to come out, Paul had been dreaming about having a cup of tea.

Widespread neglect

Unfortunately, the doctors didn't want him drinking right away, so he had to wait a few hours longer. Finally, at 8:30 pm on the 10th October, he was allowed his first cuppa. He said it was the best one he had had since the one they made him after I had given birth. He was feeling better about his legs and teeth by then and even began to joke about it. Steve came over that evening (Vanessa stayed home because she had a cold and didn't want Paul to catch that on top of everything else) and Paul kept showing him the gap in his teeth. Steve said, "now you're bald and toothless" and Paul laughed. It was a lovely sound.

That night I kissed Paul and went home at around 10:30, feeling a bit happier. I hated leaving him, he always looked so sad, but I was pleased at how the day had gone. I was always emotionally exhausted not to mention physically when I got home. I would get up at 6.00 am, shower, do a bit of housework, get together whatever I needed to take to Paul, drop Lee off at work and then be back at the hospital by 8.00 am. Despite how tired I was, I always looked forward to seeing Paul, even if he was in a miserable mood. He often was miserable in the mornings – he felt ignored during the night time, especially since a lot of nights he had trouble sleeping. Now that he was off the ventilator, he could get out of bed, but he couldn't do it on his own yet, he would have to be hoisted. Not being able to move around much made his arthritis worse during the night.

This particular morning, we were going to get him out of bed and put him on the commode for the first time, which he was really looking forward to. When I got there he was pleased to see me, despite his arthritis acting up. We sat him on the toilet and he had a movement and was thrilled to be in control of his own functions again, after having to do it in the bed or in a bedpan for so long. It's amazing how much of our own independence we take for granted. Paul was handling it very well, but it must be an awful feeling to have to wait around for people to change you as though you were a helpless infant. Especially when you are a large man and it takes four nurses just to change your bed. One of the nurses and I washed Paul when he was done in the bathroom and sat him in an armchair. He looked so happy to be sitting up like a normal person again. Doctors would pass by his window and stop and smile at him, then poke their heads in to tell him how amazing they thought he was. He would smile right back at all of them, which is surprising when you consider how much he had suffered at the hands of the NHS and that he wouldn't even have been in that position if they had cared for him properly in the first place.

As Paul sat in his chair, he asked for a cup of water to sip and he said that for the first time he felt as if he was getting better. He asked me for a kiss, which of course I was more than happy to give him. Then at dinnertime he wanted ice cream. They said I could give him a little tub and he relished every mouthful. He hadn't had any food since the 28th September and now it was the 11th October. He still had the food tube running into his nose, but it was wonderful to see him eating again. The one thing weighing on my mind that day was the state of Paul's leg and feet. A doctor had come by earlier and the look on his face frightened me. He couldn't even look Paul in the face. How much further would they have to amputate? Would my husband ever be able to walk on his own again?

That day I managed to get home for a couple of hours in the afternoon in an attempt to establish some sort of normal routine again. I didn't like leaving Paul, but the house was in a terrible mess and I wanted to make some dinner for the boys for a change. I came back to sit with Paul in the evening though, keeping him company until he fell asleep. Then I kissed him softly on the forehead, said "nite nite Paul, love you" and crept out.

Now that Paul was beginning to recover and was more aware, he began to feel the pain a lot more. The nights were especially difficult for him as I wasn't around to help him move and the nurses didn't always have time for him. Some of them were fantastic, but there were others who resented the amount of time I spent there. I didn't see how they could be opposed to a wife trying to make sure her critically ill husband was looked after, but their feelings weren't my problem anyway. Paul was my priority

Widespread neglect

and he would have all my support. Sometimes when I came in at 8.00 am, Paul would complain to me about how certain nurses had not given him the attention that he needed. I know that they have other patients to look after, but it was the ITU, which means that the patients there needed extra special care.

He had begun suffering terrible back pain and we didn't really know why. The doctors and nurses just assumed it was from sitting or laying down so much. At night he would ask the nurses to help move him to ease the pain and he told me that sometimes they would make him wait an hour or two before they came along. Of course, by then he would be in quite a state and would be difficult with them. Sometimes he would just ask to use the commode, thinking they would come more quickly and it would be a way of getting moved around. Still, it took them thirty to sixty minutes to do that. One time they got him on the commode and then left him there for two hours! He was very upset about it and when I got there, he asked me to sort it out. It was always the same nurses that he complained about. Most of the time I could calm him so that we didn't have to take it any further. It seemed to me that the nurses began to take advantage of this – they knew that even if he complained to me, I wouldn't usually make an issue of it. They didn't dare mistreat him when I was around though.

We had now reached the 12th October. It was a Thursday and I arrived at the hospital at 8.00 am as usual. We had a good, restful day talking a lot. Two doctors came by and said that if all went well, they would be able to move him out of the ITU early the following week. One of the doctors wanted him transferred to a high dependency ward, but they didn't actually have one at the hospital. The other doctor assured us that he would find the appropriate ward for Paul. They also said it would be weeks still before they knew what sort of lasting damage had been caused by the dehydration this time around. A tissue viability nurse came up to look over Paul's feet and to counsel on how they should be bandaged. It was decided that a very expensive skin-like covering would be put over the dying bits so that the flesh wouldn't be pulled off every time they rebandaged them. She showed one of the ITU nurses how to apply it properly. When she left, the ITU nurse told us that had Paul been in a Manchester hospital, this would never have happened.

"What do you mean?" I asked her, confused. Surely the doctors wouldn't have let Paul's feet get like this if there was something they could have done. She explained to us that she had done her training in a very good burns unit in Manchester and in cases where drugs or burns stopped the blood from going to the feet, they had machines that they used. These machines acted like pumps and when they were placed on the feet they would draw the blood down. Needless to say, Paul and I were quite upset to find out that with proper treatment, all the problems with Paul's feet might have been avoided. Paul's feet were still leaking large amounts of fluid and when he was sitting in his chair, sheets and towels would have to be placed under them to absorb it all. Sometimes, if someone walked nearby and wasn't looking, they would step in the fluid, which would make Paul very embarrassed. To help prevent this, the nurses put lots of absorbent padding around the bandages.

By now Paul was really fed up of being in the hospital and of not having the assistance he needed to move around, even for simple things like going to the bathroom. Some mornings when I got there, I would just have to stand there and take whatever anger he had built up over night. Not that he was abusive towards me, but he was just so frustrated from the pain and from being ignored by the nurses. I remember the next weekend being particularly trying. He wanted me to spend the night, but I was too exhausted and I didn't really get to sleep when I stayed in the hospital. I would have to promise him that I would stay so that he would calm down a bit, then sneak out after he had fallen asleep to get a few hours of sleep at home. I felt awful leaving him on his own, but there was only so much I could take myself.

In addition to his worsening back pain, Paul began to complain of difficulty in breathing, he described it as his "throat closing in." All his central lines had been taken out by this point and he was free of all the machines and drips. He was able to take his tablets orally again and was due to be moved out of the ITU that Monday 16th October. The only thing that he was still connected to was his food tube and that would come out shortly before he moved onto the ward.

Paul was put into a four-bed room and transferred from his special ITU bed to a normal hospital bed. The sister came along to welcome us, going through all of Paul's medication with the ITU nurse. The man in the bed next to us was named Kevin and he was lovely. I think he was diabetic and in his early thirties. He saw that we were both very frightened and within a few hours had offered to look after Paul for me if I needed to go home or leave for any reason.

As soon as Paul was settled into his new bed, his back started to play up again. He said the pain was unbelievable and that he had to get out of bed. So straight away I went over to the nurse and they brought the hoist to the side of his bed. They rolled him over to get the jacket underneath him, then rolled him back to the other side and hooked it up to the hoist. As they were lifting and lowering him to the floor, his gown fell open and one of the staff nurses noticed something on his back. Right above the crease in his bottom there was a big hole – a pressure sore that had gone right down to the bone. Now we knew what was most likely wrong with his back. There had been a scar there from an accident he had as a child and apparently it had opened up and not been noticed by anyone on the ITU. They left Paul there in the hoist while they documented and measured it and, though we were obviously annoyed that it had reached the state that it had, we were also relieved that we had finally found the cause of his pain and would now be able to treat it. It was cleaned, filled with a seaweed treatment and then a soft, sticky pad put over it. Of course, even though it was being treated, the pain remained the same and Paul was in extreme discomfort. I wished that that he could have remained in the ITU bed, as that was remote-controlled. He constantly wanted to be moved to alleviate the pain and couldn't do that on his own. But unfortunately the special ITU beds were needed for the patients in the ITU.

As the evening went on, Paul got more and more distressed and wanted me to stay the night with him. Now that he was out of the ITU, he would no longer have the one-to-one contact with a nurse that he was used to and was afraid that he would have to wait ages to get anything done, even during the daytime. But I was exhausted and did not want to spend another night in the hospital. I hated leaving Paul when he was so upset. But if I didn't get any rest, I would burn out.

Later that night, Paul started crying because of the pain, saying that he didn't feel safe. They had told him that they didn't even want him sitting on the edge of his bed, as he might fall out and couldn't use his feet to stop himself falling, so he had to lie on his back in pain. One of the nurses came over then and I began to explain to her how scared Paul was about the coming night and about not being able to manage under all the pain. She assured us that he would be a priority and that all he needed to do was to ring his bell and they would be there to take care of him. Kevin in the next bed said that he would ring his bell if Paul needed help and couldn't do it himself. Paul was a bit reassured and through his tears told me that it would be OK if I went home. Even so, I didn't manage to get away until midnight and called as soon as I got home to make sure that he was alright.

I felt miserable as I left that night and was crying as I walked out of the hospital. I was just glad that the day was finally over and prayed that tomorrow would be better. The next morning I woke at 5.00, showered and dressed, then tidied up around the house a bit. I was looking forward to seeing Paul and called at about 7:30 to see how his night had been. The nurse warned me on the phone that Paul had been a bit restless and when I got in at 8.00 am, he told me how horrible it had been. The bed was awful and, despite what the nurse had said the night before, they hadn't had enough time to see to him. He had wanted urine bottles, as he couldn't get out of bed to wee, and said he had waited for two hours in the night for them to bring his bottles. It still amazed me how hospital staff could ignore the basic needs of their patients in this way. Of course they were busy, but isn't this the sort of thing they were supposed to be busy doing? You don't think of it until you find yourself in the situation, but it's horribly embarrassing to have to rely on strangers for your basic bodily needs - to have to ask repeatedly really makes you lose your dignity. I felt awful for him.

Straight away I went back down the corridor and called the chief executive's office, asking to speak to the director of nursing. I told her what had been going on, saying, "Paul's just not happy. You can't treat him like this." I was so cross – what did it take to get my husband properly cared for in hospital? She said she would be right down and when she arrived, I introduced her to Paul. He had never met her before as the last time she came to see us, he had been in a coma. She told us that she had permission to hire Paul a bed similar to the one he had in the ITU and that she would speak to the sister in charge about having a representative from the bed company come in to assess Paul's needs. We then went to have a chat in private.

I was worried about how long this would all take to get sorted, as Paul was suffering in the meantime. She assured me that it would get done "ASAP" and in the meantime I thought about the chair they had given Paul. It wasn't in very good condition – the seat dipped way down in the middle and the vinyl was ripped. I thought of Paul's electric remote-controlled chair sitting at home not getting used at all and asked her if I could have that brought in for him instead. She agreed straight away, saying that they would send two porters to our house to fetch it.

I rushed back to Paul, thrilled to finally have some good news to tell him. Not only was the chair comfortable to sit in, but he could sleep in it if need be until his new bed arrived. I was sure that he would love to have something from home as well, something that was his. He smiled when I told him and that meant everything to me. He had such a lovely, cheeky smile and he was so easily pleased. Despite everything that he was going through, the thought of having something as simple as his own chair to sit in could still make him happy.

They extended the visiting hours on the ward, just for a trial period they said. Now anyone could visit from 11.00 am till 8.00 pm. The nurses didn't like it at first, as they thought it would interfere with their work. But I think they should have seen the positive side - the only people who chose to spend that much time at a hospital were those who wanted to help care for their loved ones. Every day I would wash Paul and take him to the toilet in his wheelchair, so I can't see how things like that could have been viewed as interference.

During my time there, when I had the opportunity to concentrate on something other than Paul, I saw quite a few bad things happen. Nothing criminal, but just repeated instances of poor patient care. Every day there was someone on the ward who was unhappy with the way they were being treated. Many patients, particularly the elderly, wouldn't complain because then they knew they would be treated worse by the staff for making a fuss. I felt so bad for them, as they were totally dependent on these people and didn't deserve to be treated the way they were.

Paul's chair was brought in and his bed arrived not too long after. It was an air bed with remote control, so now Paul could move without having to call for the nurses. I tried my best to look after his basic needs, so that slowly he began to regain his dignity and strength. We settled into life on the ward quite well. Kevin, in the next bed, went home after a few days and another lovely man called Patrick arrived. He suffered from rheumatoid arthritis and diabetes like Paul, as well as having pretty bad asthma. Like me, his wife would come in first thing in the morning to wash and dress him. All in all, things seemed to be getting better for us.

The main concern now was Paul's feet and left leg. The doctors were waiting to see if they would get better before deciding how much to amputate. They were being dressed every other day at this point and the smell was not as bad as before. The blistering on the left calf had almost gone and it was healing nicely. The foot was still horrible though – it started right under the ball of the foot and went right down to every toe, except for one small island of healthy flesh just under his big toe. The doctors hoped that, because that one piece just about an inch in diameter had remained healthy, the areas around it might recover and then they would just have to remove part of the foot instead of the lower leg. They were optimistic, but also doubtful. Some of the toes on his left foot had gone rock hard, they were like stone when you tapped them. They had thought at one stage that the right foot might heal entirely, but it had not. All of the toes were now dead and would need to be removed, as well as a small portion of the foot. Every day four physio girls would come over. They had arranged a time to meet on the ward to get Paul standing. Paul really looked forward to this bit of independence, I suppose it made him feel whole again and not disabled. He was laughing a lot more now too – Patrick, at the side of him, was a very funny man. Sometimes it seemed we spent the whole day laughing.

My routine was better now as well. I felt as if I was getting everything done that I needed to and I didn't worry about the boys or the housework so much anymore. Every day I would get up at 6:30, shower and do my hair, then do some housework. After that I would get the boys up and make them some tea and breakfast if they were lucky. At 7.00, I would make my morning call to the hospital to see how Paul had been during the night. Assuming that everything had gone well, I would see to Sheba, then collect anything that Paul needed for that day – clean boxers and towels, etc. – and make quick calls to his mum and mine to let them know what was going on. I would drop Lee off at work on my way to the hospital, where I usually arrived around 8.00. Paul would get extra toast with his breakfast and would have some waiting for me when I got there. Then I would sit down and relax for a bit while eating with him.

After his breakfast, I would get a bowl and all of his things, pull the curtain around his bed, wash him and change his clothes. We would then wait for the hoist to be brought around so I could get him out of bed and onto the commode. Then it was on to his chair to wait for the physio girls and the dressing of his leg and feet. We would read the papers to pass the time until lunch and any doctors who were doing rounds would normally come then as well. Depending on what I had to do that day, I would sometimes ask Paul if he minded me going home at around 3:30 for a couple of hours to make dinner for the boys. He never liked it, but he knew that they needed me too. He would always tell me to please hurry back and I would.

So I would go home and do whatever odd jobs needed doing, make Paul a couple of sandwiches and put together a few treats for him, then make dinner for the boys. I would collect Lee from work and drop him off at home, but Adam had a van from his job, so he could drive himself home. At 5:30 pm, I would leave to go back to Paul and arrive just as dinner was being sorted out for the patients. Then I would stay until midnight. Every night before I left, I would make sure that he had everything that he needed at hand, like urine bottles and water jugs. I didn't want him to have to wait for hours if he needed anything and experience had already taught me that you couldn't always rely on the nurses, who had a lot of other patients to care for. As I left, I would look back at Paul and he would smile at me and tell me not to be late in the morning. As I walked along the long corridors at night on my way home, I would sometimes run into the night-shift staff coming back from their breaks. They would laugh at me for still being there and jokingly ask me, "don't you have a home to go to?" To be honest, I didn't really feel like I did, because without Paul, it wasn't home. So we made the best out of a bad situation and made the hospital our home.

I was very watchful of Paul and now that he was more aware, he was quite careful as well. Even though he still couldn't move to take care of himself, he would fill in his own fluid charts every day and make sure he drank and passed enough water. I spent so much time there, that I had plenty of opportunity to observe how the staff interacted with the patients, Paul and others. Some of the nurses on the ward were lovely, but there were others who were just plain miserable. Most patients would ignore a nurse who was grumpy or snapped at them and some of them even had a

Widespread neglect

laugh together behind the nurses' backs. But others would feel intimidated and sometimes snap back themselves, particularly the elderly. Of course that would only make everything worse. The nurses themselves were aware of this problem – I remember some of the good nurses confiding in me that they worried about what would happen if one of their loved ones had to go into hospital, because they saw the sort of abuse that went on daily. Many of the nurses would scold their patients or leave them waiting for ages when they asked for basic things. Some of them were so unpleasant when they spoke to the patients, particularly the elderly, that I would feel ashamed. One time I actually intervened and told a male nurse to leave and that I would deal with the gentleman whom he had been telling off. The nurse had restrained the man by holding his hands down very tightly when he wouldn't do as he was told. The patient was about eighty years old and of course he became frightened at this and even more difficult. I could see that he wasn't exactly being agreeable, but that still didn't mean he needed to be physically restrained.

There was one man brought onto the ward with a chest infection that was complicated by a heart bypass done some months earlier. When he came in, he was walking and eating and getting out of bed on his own, but as the days went on, all of this stopped. I began to get worried because it's when you become so dependent on other people for your basic needs that things start to go wrong. He was being helped to wash, but no one was paying attention to what he ate or drank. Whatever was given to him was later removed and then documented as "refused by patient," which was a blatant lie. He was too weak to eat or drink, much less refuse anything. His fluids weren't being monitored at all and, as far as I could see, he hadn't had anything to drink for three days. After all that had gone on with Paul, I couldn't stand it. I went to the sister and told her that the man had not had anything to drink for days. She said that she would sort it out. They moved him to a different room later that afternoon. He was still on the same ward though, so I watched his family as they came and went over the next few days, looking more and more worried. Four days later he died of heart and kidney failure. I saw his family after they were told of his death. They were huddled together crying. Of course they didn't know enough to question why his heart and kidneys had failed, they just assumed that it was natural for that to happen. But he had only come in with a chest infection. I was sure that he had died from dehydration.

As time went on, I saw several other patients die in a similar way. I had become particularly close to one of the nurses and I when I asked her about it, she told me that they called it "hospital syndrome". While we were on that ward, whenever anyone died in those circumstances, she would come to me and say, "Mandy, we lost another one last night with hospital syndrome." It was abuse, plain and simple, even though there was no physical or verbal violence involved. These patients, who were too weak or unaware to complain or ask for things themselves, were being deprived of food and water. Of course, they were handed them, but what good did that do when they couldn't feed or drink on their own? I was shocked and vowed never to leave Paul alone in a hospital again.

I became disgusted with some of the nurses, who didn't seem to be bothered by any of this at all. They were always hiding behind the excuses of staff shortages and blaming the administration or the management or the government. And the administration and government were to blame in a way – for allowing this to go on. But the truth of the matter is that many of these nurses just did not care for their patients. There were many good nurses as well and I am by no means trying to say that all hospital staff are uncaring. Many of them were loving people who went into the medical profession so that they could help others. But you have to be careful and if your loved one has to go into hospital, you have to make sure that they are properly looked after. You mustn't assume that they will be taken care of just because the staff have medical training or that they always know what they are doing. If you are concerned about something, you shouldn't be afraid to voice it, even if the doctors or nurses try to make you feel

Widespread neglect

as though you don't know what you are talking about. Paul and I had learned these lessons the hard way.

One of the senior doctors came around to visit Paul a few days after he came onto the ward, bringing eight or nine medical students with him. The doctor introduced the students to Paul and then called a nurse over and asked her to remove the bandages from Paul's feet and left leg. Everyone gathered around and you could see the expressions on the young doctors' faces turn to horror and then sympathy as they glanced up at Paul. The senior doctor started explaining to them what had happened to Paul. He told them that Paul's condition had resulted from his diabetes, as though this was a normal consequence of the disease. I wasn't sure if I should say anything, but finally I couldn't take it any more.

"Excuse me," I said, "I don't like to interrupt you when you are talking to your students, but this did not happen to Paul because of his diabetes. It happened because he was dehydrated in the hospital and went into renal failure due to a chemical imbalance. He then had to be put on life support, including noradrenalin, which is a vascular restrictor. That cut off the blood supply and that's what happened to his legs."

The doctor just stood there staring at me and then looked at the students. They all seemed quite embarrassed and were standing there waiting for him to say something. His eyes were very angry when he turned back to me and asked, "who told you this? No one confirmed that to me."

"Speak to any of the doctors," I replied, "it wasn't his diabetes."

He apologised and left with all his students. I was incredibly cross. Did he really think we were that stupid? Did they do this regularly to people – try to convince them that their illnesses are perfectly normal, when they are actually a result of hospital neglect? I suppose most people are afraid to contradict doctors, but there was no way I was going to allow him to cover up what had happened. Those students were tomorrow's doctors and would soon have patients of their own. They deserved to be told the truth, so that what had happened to Paul wouldn't happen to anyone else.

The doctor couldn't look me in the face after that. Before he left, he came back into the room to tell Paul that he would be back to see him the next week. He only looked at Paul, never once at me. I think he disliked me very much, but that wasn't something I was going to lose sleep over. Later on that day, Paul laughed about the whole affair, but I was still fuming. A nurse came over a short while later to redress Paul's feet and said to me softly, "you're a very brave lady". The word had got out already, apparently. That hadn't been my intention, I had just wanted to make sure that those students knew the truth. There was a male nurse, with whom we become quite close. I was speaking to him later that day about what had happened and he told me not to worry. "I looked into Paul's file," he said, "and everything is documented in there. They know that you had to ask to have his fluid balance monitored and all of that, so no one can claim that all this is a result of his diabetes." I was relieved to hear all of this. It would certainly come in handy later.

A few days after the incident with the doctor, I went home in the afternoon to get some housework done. Paul was feeling reasonably comfortable and wanted to get some sleep, so I thought I would take advantage of the time. He had had a cough for a few days, but other than that, his condition remained more or less the same. It was about 5:30 pm when the phone at home rang. I had collected Lee from work, finished doing dinner for the boys and was just about to get ready to go back to the hospital. It was the man in the bed opposite Paul's. By now they all knew his story and had agreed to watch out for him when I wasn't there and let me know if anything bad happened.

"Mandy," he said to me, "Paul asked me to call you. You had better come quickly." My heart dropped, but he must have realised how nervous I would be, so then he said, "don't worry too much, but they have given Paul the wrong medication and he asked me to ring you to come back in straight away as he is scared and can't breath very well." I arrived to find Paul very anxious, but

68

Widespread neglect

otherwise OK. One of the nurses came over to us to explain what had happened. She told us that there was a lady on the ward who needed to be sedated because she was screaming all the time. Her medication had been on the trolley along with Paul's linctus for his cough. They were in similar bottles and the nurse had accidentally administered the sedative to Paul. As soon as he drank it, he mentioned that it tasted different. She looked at the label and realised her mistake immediately. She called a doctor right away, who checked Paul over and said that he had to be monitored every hour for that night, as sedatives can cause respiratory problems. The doctor assured me that Paul would be fine though and that they were just taking precautions.

As time went on, it became obvious that the sedative had not done any serious or lasting damage to Paul. The other patients on the ward said they could not believe Paul's luck. I was very glad that he had mentioned that the medicine tasted different, because if he hadn't, they might never have spotted their mistake or known to monitor him. In the worst case, had Paul died during the night, everybody would have just assumed he had died from his illnesses rather than from being given the wrong medicine.

Chapter 6

The amputations

Every day as the nurses put new dressings on Paul's legs, it became obvious that they were deteriorating. The pain was increasing, but Paul did not want to overdo the painkillers, as he was worried about how his kidneys would cope with all the drugs after all that they had been through. I think that deep down, Paul knew that he would have to have his leg amputated, but he tried to remain optimistic. I overheard him one day telling his sister that he hoped it could be saved. I was glad that he was still positive. But I didn't want him to have any false hopes, so I sat down and told him that it was not a matter of whether or not they would amputate, but how much they would have to take off.

The way that one doctor had explained it to us was that there was a chance that some of the blood supply would be able to get through. If it did, then the blackness should draw back and the leg begin to heal. In that case, he would only have to take most of the foot and would be able to leave the heel on the left leg. This was important, because if you can keep the heel, then you can still balance with a weighted shoe. But if there wasn't enough of the heel left, then the leg would have to come off below the knee. Also, in order to keep the heel, there had to be enough healthy skin left to fold over the end of the amputation and that wasn't looking very likely in Paul's case. With the right foot, we already knew that all of the toes would have to come off and possibly part of the foot.

I don't remember the exact date, but somewhere around the 6th or 7th November, they made the decision on Paul's left leg. When the nurse came to dress the leg that day, she took off the

The amputations

bandages and said to me, "what do you think Mandy?" I looked at the foot and it was obvious to both of us that it was becoming infected. She left the leg out of the bandages and put in a call to the surgeon. He came around later that day to look at the foot. The dead piece was coming apart from the healthy bit, as though it were being pushed away, and there were signs of infection. He looked up at Paul and said, "I'm sorry, but it has to come off below the knee. You're going to lose your leg."

I was standing behind Paul, holding him around his shoulders. I don't think I could have faced looking at him just then. I could feel him trembling and my lip started to quiver, but I didn't dare cry, because I was afraid that I wouldn't be able to stop. As the surgeon left, one of the nurses came in. When she saw us, she asked me the question with her eyes and I nodded yes. She started to cry and when Paul saw that, it set him off too. He put his head in his hands and broke down. She hugged him tightly and said, "you're so brave." I held him then too and said "it'll be fine, don't cry, please." His tears hurt me so much that I didn't think I would be able to stand it. She backed off to give us time to get over the news and to try to compose herself as well. I made Paul lift his head up and said to him, "this won't stop you Paul, you're so strong. You'll get a new leg and you'll walk again, you know you will." We kissed and hugged and kept on crying. I kept thinking, 'why us? Why is all this happening to us?' But I still hoped that maybe things would get better, that this would be the worst of it and that after the amputation, we could look forward to moving on.

Over the course of the next few days, they began to prepare us for the amputation, explaining the procedure and what we could expect. They wanted Paul to go back to the ITU a few days before the operation. That way, if any problems arose, they would be better able to deal with them. The operation would be done with the aid of an epidural, but they would begin the epidural a few days before the procedure itself. The epidural was necessary because a general anaesthetic was too risky for someone in Paul's condition.

The operation was scheduled for the 20th November. Paul would go back to the ITU on the 17th and the epidural would be

The amputations

inserted on the 18th. We still had a few days to get used to the idea of losing the leg. During those days, Paul and I talked about what would happen when his leg was removed. It had become a horrible mess and, though the idea of losing it was extremely painful, it would also be a relief not to have to deal with it anymore. I knew that he would recover. He was a strong man and I felt humbled by him because he was so brave. The physio talked to us about getting Paul a new leg. Paul had a lot of respect for her and she told him of many young men about his age who were up and walking again on new limbs in no time. Despite the odds, things began to look positive again. We were both looking forward to resuming our normal lives, outside of the hospital, finally. We felt as though our lives had been put on hold since May the previous year, when Paul was first dehydrated. For a year and a half, we had been controlled by one medical condition after another and we just wanted to go back to normal. We wanted to return to our home, our sons, our dogs and our friends.

Paul's breathing was still not good and he couldn't seem to get rid of the cough that had been bothering him, though they continued giving him the linctus. One night he started coughing as though something were caught in his throat. It went on for a long time and his breathing was very laboured that night. The nurses asked the anaesthetist from the ITU to come down and have a look. After he examined Paul, he said that most likely it was a stridor. I had no idea what that was, so he explained to me that it was scarring in the windpipe caused by the ventilator, so the linctus they were giving Paul had been of no use. He said that it should heal itself in time, so we didn't get too worried. Since Paul was scheduled to go back to the ITU, he said that he would ask the director of medicine at the hospital to have a look at Paul and maybe do a bronchoscope (look down the throat with a camera) to confirm his assessment.

The days went by and Paul went back to the ITU. This time he was put into one of the beds in the main room, which held six patients. We could see people coming and going and this made it

The amputations

less lonely for us. We had got to know lots of people during Paul's stay in the hospital and many of them came to wish him well that day. It seemed as if he was being kissed or having his hand shaken all day long.

The next day the 18th November, Paul went to the theatre to have his epidural inserted. He said that it had hurt a little, but that he felt fine and that his legs were beginning to go numb. Paul had asked Adam and Lee if they would take the day off work on the 20th, so that they could be with me while he was in surgery. I insisted that I would be fine, but for some reason he wanted us all together. He confessed to me the night before that he was afraid he might not make it and wanted to see his sons again. I started crying. I felt awful and assured him that he would be fine and that he shouldn't even be thinking that way. Of course nothing could take the thoughts out of his head, so we just sat talking for the rest of the evening, with me trying to calm and soothe him. I finally left at around midnight, after he had fallen asleep.

The next morning the three of us arrived at the hospital around 7:30 am. Paul was awake and anxious and began crying when he saw us. I hugged him and told him that I loved him. My stomach was turning inside out, so I can't imagine what he must have been feeling, not to mention the two boys. At about 11.00 am, they came to take him for the bronchoscope. Paul mentioned to them that he had started to feel his legs again and they said that they would sort that out after the bronchoscope. We sat and waited around his bed space. They came back at about 1:30 pm and apparently all had gone well with the first procedure. However, for some reason the epidural had failed, so they decided to go ahead with the amputation using local anaesthetic along with a sedative to help Paul forget. We didn't really have much time to think about it, because soon they were back to take him to the theatre again. Adam and Lee were so frightened as they sat by their father's bed and all three men had to fight to keep the tears back. As the assistants began pulling Paul's bed out of its space to take him for the amputation, he held his hand out and shook his sons' hands, saying "it's been nice knowing you both." His face was white and

74

The amputations

Adam and Lee both had to turn away because they couldn't keep the tears back any longer. His words crushed me.

I walked with him to the doors, which was as far as I was allowed to go. I could hardly see for all the tears, but I was trying hard to be brave and not get hysterical. When we got to the door, we were stopped by the assistants, who suddenly realised that Paul had not signed a consent form for the operation. It should have been signed some days before, but had somehow been overlooked. Paul completely broke down now and sat in his bed sobbing inconsolably. All I could do was hold him until the surgeon came from the theatre with a consent form for him to sign. It said that he gave them permission to amputate below his knee on his left leg and all the toes and the forefoot of the right leg. He was still crying as he signed it. Nearby, I could see three nurses standing watching us. They had come to say good luck, but decided against it as we were all so distressed. They were crying too. As they began moving him again, I kissed him and told him that I loved him and would see him soon. The boys hadn't been able to face watching their father getting carted off again, so they had gone out for a walk. All I could do was sit by Paul's bed space and wait for him to be brought back. I sat near the window and watched people going about their business in the hospital. At one point a doctor came in to tell me that the bronchoscope showed that there had been damage to Paul's throat, but that it should heal on its own. I thanked him and then went back to watching people.

After Paul had been in surgery for a couple of hours, the ITU doctor came out and told me that Paul was fine and the operation was going well. He said that they were about halfway through. Steve and Vanessa arrived at some point and some others from my family. At about 7:15 pm the theatre doors opened and out came Paul, awake. I ran over and hugged him, saying "see stupid, you're alive!" He was crying again, but this time because he was so happy he had made it through. Then I looked down and saw the empty space where his leg used to be. Somehow, it shocked me. Even after all the talking and thinking we had done about his leg being amputated, I was unprepared for the sight of it.

The amputations

I think I lost control then. I went over to a nurse and begged her to take him back to the theatre and sew the leg back on. I kept saying to her, "I don't care if it's black and dead, we'll live with it and I'll make it better, just please sew it back on!" She took me to a side room and made me a cup of tea. "That's not going to happen," she said softly, trying to calm me with her voice. "You have been so brave throughout all of this and so supportive and now he needs you more than ever."

I don't know how, but eventually I pulled myself together. I knew Paul would be wondering where I was and why I had left him at a time like this. I was so glad that I had managed not to break down in front of him. I shuddered when I thought how awful it would have made him feel if, on top of having to deal with losing his leg, he had heard his wife begging the nurse to sew it back on. I went back to his bedside and thought he looked pretty good considering he'd just had a major operation. He was still on the drips and was connected to a morphine pump. The rest of the night went by in a bit of a blur for me. I remember talking to Paul for hours. He didn't want to let me go and he deserved to have whatever he wanted. It was about 1.00 am by the time I got out of there that night and I still don't know if I really believed that Paul's leg was gone forever.

Next day I arrived bright and early at 8.00 am. Paul was smiling at me and I smiled back. Normally I would wash him at this point, but I didn't want to lift up the sheets. I had been dreading it all night. I knew the leg would be bandaged, but I was still too scared to look. I tried not to show this though and eventually worked up the nerve to do what I had to do. There was a drain inserted at the side of the leg to take away any excess blood and waste, but the rest of it was in bandages, as well as his right foot. He was in a little pain, but nothing he couldn't deal with. Most of all, he was just glad to be alive.

The physio came over to show him how he should be exercising his legs and, though it was difficult for him to move, he tried his best. She stressed the importance of the exercises, as then the wound would heal faster and the muscles strengthen more

76

The amputations

quickly. True to form, by the end of that first day Paul had mastered the exercises and was moving his legs around quite freely. After that, the physio came by twice a day to see how Paul was doing and she was very pleased with his progress. I tried to behave normally though I was still in shock. Strangely enough, Paul seemed to be dealing with it better than I was and was in fine spirits. Somehow I think he sensed that I needed him to be strong for me. He was a celebrity too – all the doctors and nurses kept coming over to tell him how brave they thought he was. "You're amazing!" I heard them say to him over and over that day.

They only wanted to keep Paul in the ITU for a few days, because they thought it would get depressing for him seeing so much death after being so near it himself. Not many people come out of the ITU alive, so I suppose Paul had been one of the lucky ones. They planned to remove the drain from his stump after three days and, assuming that all went well, transfer him onto a ward after five. There wasn't much blood being drained away, but taking it out turned out to be more troublesome than I had thought. A nurse had to pull the tube out of the hole punched into Paul's knee. Paul was terrified that it might hurt and of course that made her nervous as well. She began by pulling the curtains around the bed and then peeled back the bandages. She asked Paul if he could feel anything and he said yes and that it hurt. She tried for about fifteen minutes to pull it out without causing him any pain, but didn't get very far. Paul was worried that his leg would get ripped open and the nurse was worried about causing him too much pain. Eventually the physio came by. By then, I couldn't stand it any more. "Why don't we hold you?" I said to Paul, "and then Sally can pull it out all in one go and be done with it." He agreed and we each held on to one of his hands, blocking his view of the nurse with our bodies. The physio told him that he could scream as loud as he wanted if that helped and he took her up on it. When the nurse pulled the cord out, he let out a solid yell and I held him close until the pain was gone. A few moments later I went outside the curtains and all the ITU nurses were standing around watching. "It's a girl," I said and they all smiled.

The amputations

Paul was moved out of the ITU and back to the ward on the 26th November. He seemed to recover amazingly quickly from the amputations, so the next thing on our minds was when we would be able to go home. He had been there nine weeks already and was desperate to get out. First the occupational therapists would need to see our house though, to make sure that Paul would be able to get around easily. Luckily we had a downstairs bedroom and bathroom, so the only real problem would be actually getting him in and out of the house.

One thing that they had to make sure of, before they let him come home, was that he could move himself around well enough from bed to wheelchair and wheelchair to toilet, etc. Knowing this, he worked very hard at it and by the following week the therapists agreed to take Paul home on a visit to see how he could get around on his own there. But first the bandages had to come off. When the day came to peel the dressing off, I could barely look and stood there with my hands over my eyes, peeking through my fingers. I expected there to be lots of cuts and blood. When the nurse got all the bandages off, I was relieved. All you could see was a line, like a pencil mark, around the end of the stump on one leg and the end of the foot on the other. We were both amazed at how good it looked, though I couldn't bring myself to touch it just yet. Seeing the empty space where his leg and foot used to be still broke my heart.

The surgeon came in the next day to look at Paul's legs and was pleased not only with the way the wounds were healing, but also by how adept Paul had become at moving himself around. He agreed that Paul was just about ready for a home visit and hopefully they could release him soon after. There had been a point, not that long before, when I had thought I might never take Paul home again, so this was great news. As he was leaving though, the surgeon had some surprising and disturbing news for us. "Oh, by the way, I had a dream about you last night," he said to Paul, turning back from the door. "I woke up and was still thinking about you and then I finally realised that I forgot to send a piece of your leg to pathology to be analysed. I'm sorry, but I had it

The amputations

destroyed." I was stunned, but since I wasn't really sure what was going on, I decided not to say anything right there and then. But I remembered (and had also noted in my diary) him asking his senior house officer the day of the amputation to send a piece of Paul's leg to pathology to be examined – was it possible that both doctors had forgotten something as routine as sending a sample of an amputated limb over to pathology? Or were they trying to hide something? This was the doctor that had tried convincing Paul, me and the medical students that Paul's diabetes was to blame for his amputations. The amputated leg was the only physical proof that the problems with Paul's legs had been caused in the hospital and not by his diabetes. Would they simply get rid of the evidence, rather than admitting that Paul had not had vein or leg disease caused by his diabetes? The nurses had told us that the amputation was a result of his legs being deprived of blood from the noradrenalin when he was on life support. And Paul had only been on life support because he had gone into a coma after being discharged in renal failure. All this worried me. Moreover, I couldn't get out of my head what one nurse had said about the hospital in Manchester and how Paul would still have had his legs if he had been treated there instead.

Paul was progressing wonderfully and was going to the gym for physio and building up his body. Now that he was feeling better, he was joking with everyone and causing havoc and it was lovely to see him laughing with the nurses and other patients. Don't get me wrong, it wasn't exactly a bed of roses, but there was a lot of optimism and it began to look as if we would be able to get our lives back on track. Obviously things would never be as they had been, but maybe they could be almost as good.

There was a volunteer who would come on the ward every day to make an afternoon cup of tea for the patients, a man named Ken. He was in his seventies but very active and you could see that he really enjoyed talking to all of the patients. Paul got along quite well with him and looked forward to seeing him every day. Ken came in one day after Paul had gone for his physio and nodded at me from over behind the kitchen door. That meant "I've done you

The amputations

a cuppa." I nodded back, which meant, "yes, thank you." He walked over with the tea, still stirring it and stood by my side, saying, "Paul is always so funny and happy. He's an inspiration considering he's an amputee." I just smiled back at him. "Everyone is talking about a man in this hospital at the moment who has lost both his legs due to a mistake that the hospital made," Ken continued.

"Really?" I asked, "that's awful!"

"Well, it's true," he said. "Wouldn't it be wonderful if Paul could talk to this man, show him how amputees can still smile and laugh?" I agreed, but Ken said that he didn't know the man's name or even which ward he was on, but that he would try to find out and let me know. Then he went off on his rounds. When Ken left, one of my favourite nurses came over and smiled at me, saying, "I couldn't help overhearing your conversation. Didn't you realise?"

"Realise what?" I asked.

"The man Ken was on about was Paul!" she said.

I was stunned, but then thinking back to the conversation, realised that of course she was right. I had been thrown for a moment by Ken saying that the man had lost both legs, but I suppose people tend to generalise. I found it interesting that the general feeling seemed to be that Paul's amputations had been due to hospital neglect and that everyone was talking about it.

Chapter 7

Coming home

The day for the home visit was planned and I was asked not to come in to the hospital that morning because they wanted to see how Paul coped with washing and dressing himself. They had to see for themselves what his needs were, in order to determine if he would be able to function on his own at home. They arrived at our house at around 11:30 am. Paul was very emotional – it had been thirteen weeks since he was last home. It took some time to get him in the front door, as the step is quite steep. Three men were needed, but eventually it was done. Paul asked to be left alone to sit there for a while, just to have a look around. Of course he didn't get any peace, because Sheba came running over, crazy with excitement because she was so happy to see her dad again.

When Paul had been in hospital, every night when I came home Sheba would go over to my bag and take Paul's dirty clothes out so she could walk around with them for a while. She had known he was alive, but must have been quite confused and worried as to why he wasn't home. I didn't mind her taking his clothes. I felt it helped her remember him and this was the only contact she had with him. Now he was home, she kept sniffing around his leg, realising that something was different and from that day on she became very protective of him, as if realising that now he needed extra special care.

The physios went through the ground floor of the house with Paul, to make sure that he would be able to get around with minimal assistance. They took him into the bathroom to watch him use the shower and toilet, then into the bedroom to see him get in and out of bed. All in all, they were quite pleased and said that

Coming home

Paul could come home, though some slight changes would need to be made. A ramp would need to be put up so that he could get in and out of the house and we would need rails in the downstairs bathroom. But these were relatively minor problems and he could come home before they were done. In the meantime, they would contact our occupational therapist and have her sort out what we would need. December 6th was the date set for his release.

The 6th finally arrived and I went to the hospital that morning feeling so many different emotions at the thought of finally bringing Paul home. Of course I was happy, excited and relieved, but I was also slightly nervous. How would Paul get along without his leg and feet? And before I could even get him home, there was one more thing that we would have to deal with – a meeting I had requested with the hospital chief executive and the director of nursing.

They had not come back to me after the last meeting, which we had held while Paul was in a coma. I had assumed that they would have done some investigating and would have something to report back to me when we met this time. I was sadly mistaken. They came down to the ward around noon and the four of us went into a staff room. Paul was introduced to them (Paul had never met the chief executive until now) and then there was silence. I had expected them to do the talking, but since they didn't, I started to. I told them that I believed that Paul had been dehydrated for a third time, even after I had written to them asking for help. I told them the names of all the doctors who had been involved and brought them up to date on everything that had happened since we last met. Paul didn't say much – I think he was too excited at the thought of going home. When I finished talking, the chief executive told me that they would look into it and asked if it would be alright if they called me in for a meeting in January. I agreed to that as the holidays were coming up. But I was very disappointed at the meeting - I didn't see that it had much point to it at all.

We went back to Paul's bed to collect his things and to say goodbye to everyone. We gave the nurses flowers and chocolates and thanked them for all the help they had given us. They all kissed Paul and wished us the best. One of the doctors passed by as we were getting ready and he stopped to have a brief chat with us. We were still worried about the stridor, but he was confident that it would settle down. He warned Paul that anxiety makes it worse and told him, if he had difficulty breathing, to try to relax and stay calm. Paul's response was, "easier said than done when you can't breathe". But he wasn't worrying much about it now, because he was so happy to be going home.

We went to the car and I managed to get Paul in safely. It was a bit difficult to see during the drive home because of all the tears in my eyes. I couldn't believe that I was finally bringing my husband back home with me after the nightmare that we had been through. As we pulled up in the driveway, I thought of how wonderful it would be not to have to get up at 6:30 every morning to go to the hospital anymore. I got Paul into the wheelchair and pushed him up to the front door. The chair was a manual one with very small wheels, but I doubted if Paul could have wheeled himself at this stage even if it had large ones. I had asked about getting an electric chair in the hospital, but we were told that the request had to go through social services. In other words, it would most likely be some time before we could hope to get one, if ever.

I unlocked our front door and then spent the next five minutes trying to get Paul through it. I didn't think I would be able to manage it at one point, but finally I got him in. It nearly killed me doing it the first time and Paul liked to go out a lot. That made me realise that I had to get the ramp sorted quickly. Paul looked around the house – this time it was just the two of us, without all the hospital staff – and then kissed me. "Thank you for all the support you gave me in the hospital," he said. "It was a pleasure," I replied, "I love you."

That evening I cooked him his favourite dinner – roast rib of beef. It was a beautiful day and although we had a difficult path ahead of us, it seemed as if we had come through the worst of it.

As we settled down to bed that night, I had a nervous feeling in the pit of my stomach. When we had been in the hospital, all I had to do when something went wrong was call one of the nurses, but now Paul was all my responsibility. I suppose that most people coming out of the hospital after a long stay would feel that way, but that doesn't make the feeling any less real. I was worried about his breathing, which still sounded very harsh and ragged. I tried to calm myself by remembering that they had chosen to discharge him and wouldn't have done so if they thought he was still in danger. Besides, the district nurses had been contacted and they would come in each day starting the next day. Paul's stump and foot still needed to be dressed and cleaned daily and, at least for the time being, they would be seeing to that. If there were any difficulties, I was sure they would be able to help me out in the morning. Still, I was nervous.

Paul had difficulty breathing that night and I kept having to get out of bed to find things to prop him up with. The flatter he was, the more problems he had getting air. But we got through it and the next morning we faced our first day together in our new circumstances. Paul was almost totally reliant on me at this stage, which didn't sit well with him at all. I tried to reassure him that he wasn't a burden and that I loved caring for him, but he had always been an independent person. That morning I got him out of bed and into his wheelchair, then pushed him to the lounge so I could help him into his armchair. Although he hated being an invalid, he was also afraid of being left alone because of his breathing. He had the perfectly rational fear of suffocating and, if no one was near him, of dying before anyone even realised that something was wrong. He didn't even want me to go upstairs while he still had the stridor. I felt that things would get better, so for the time being I decided that I would just stay with him if he wanted me to and see how things went later on.

I was glad to see the nurse when she came later that day. I felt that I really needed a bit of support. She helped me sort out Paul's medicine and over the next few days showed me how to take care of Paul's leg and foot. The right foot had healed well, but we had some slight problems with the stump of the left leg. A tiny bit of tendon was left sticking out after the surgery, so it hadn't quite healed properly and would leak. We were worried about infection, but I kept it very clean and dressed it every day.

I tried to make Paul as self-reliant as possible, for both our sakes. He had a file for his pills to keep them organised for seven days. I would make sure that it was filled up and put it on a coffee table near his chair, so that he could take his pills at the right time and wouldn't have to ask me. He had been given a nebulizer and some masks at the hospital to bring home with him and I also put those at his side. The nebulizer helped to keep his windpipe moist with saline solution, which helped his breathing. It was a lot like holding a cloth over your head and leaning over a bowl of steaming water. If ever he felt he couldn't breathe, he would just have to switch that on and put the saline in.

Despite all my efforts, over the next eleven days, Paul's health got drastically worse. His breathing became more and more difficult. The constant feeling that he was suffocating terrified him and I'm sure that made it even worse still. The doctors had told me that his condition would settle, so I kept telling him that. Then he would get angry at me and we would argue, which did not help his breathing at all. When I look back on all this I feel so guilty. I just didn't understand what he was going through at the time. For someone who has never had trouble breathing, it is difficult to grasp how terrifying it can be to feel you are not getting enough air and he had to live with it all the time. When he had bad spells, his breaths would come out in tiny little gasps and I would try my best to calm him. Sometimes it wouldn't work and then I would get scared and cross and say things like, "stop it, or else you're going to end up back in the hospital." I'm so ashamed when I think of things like that now.

By this time, the district nurse had arranged for Paul to have oxygen at home and the hospital had referred him to an ear, nose and throat (ENT) doctor. I contacted his surgery immediately and spoke to the secretary, explaining Paul's medical problems to her. I was told that Paul would have to wait his turn, just like everyone else. Like the hospital doctors, she didn't seem very worried by what I was describing.

One particularly bad night, we both ended up crying – Paul because he couldn't breathe and me because I was so scared. Crying had become something we did quite frequently. "Paul, let's call the hospital," I begged, but he refused. He desperately did not want to go back and I think that even though he was scared, he also

Coming home

believed what the doctors had told him about his condition gradually stabilising. I set the oxygen mask over his face, but I couldn't stand to see the pain in his eyes. We couldn't understand how we had got into this awful situation nor why or how the hospital had allowed it to happen. Once he had settled down, he pulled off the mask and began crying again. He could hardly speak, but when he could he said, "I don't want to die. Not after all that I have just been through and survived. I want to see my grandchildren, Mandy." I didn't know what to say. I knew I couldn't promise him that he would live to see his grandchildren, as much as I wanted it to be true. So I just held him and promised that I would try to sort things out the next day.

We had planned a homecoming party for the 16th December at Paul's Uncle Mick's and Auntie June's pub in Longford. I was worried about how Paul would cope, but I checked with the medical staff and they said it would be alright. He didn't have a fever or infection, so as long as someone was there to take him home when he got tired, everything should be fine. When we got there and I saw the look on Paul's face as he saw all the people who had come out to wish him well, I stopped worrying. I knew this party would do him much more good than harm. I had invited some of the nurses from the hospital, but most of the people were family and friends. We were both touched that so many people had cared enough to come out and see him.

Paul's mum and sister were there, which really made his night, even though they didn't say all that much to him. Two of his three little nieces, Kirsty and Charlotte, were there as well, which he was very pleased about. It was Charlotte's birthday and we had a card for her, but she wouldn't come to Paul to take it. He was upset that they were afraid of the way he looked, but he tried not to show it. He felt that, if they had been allowed to visit him regularly, they would have got used to the changes in his appearance as they happened, the way the rest of the children in the family had. My brother Stefan and his children had been frequent visitors, as had my sister Rebecca and hers, and none of them were frightened of Paul. He enjoyed them being inquisitive and would

Coming home

let them look at and touch his wounds if they wanted to, so that they wouldn't be scared. He loved children and wanted to make them at ease with his disabilities so they could still enjoy being around him. Still, these were minor setbacks and Paul really enjoyed himself that night. To say it was like old times would be lying, but we both felt that we were making the best of our lives as they were. I was proud of Paul for being able to celebrate after all he had been through.

Paul's breathing continued to worsen. I called the district nurse again. "He can't go on like this," I said, "can't we see the ENT consultant a bit earlier?" She called to see if we could get an earlier appointment, but all we were told was that it wasn't possible, so if Paul couldn't breathe, we should bring him in to casualty. I couldn't leave Paul alone for even a few seconds now, because he was so afraid that he would die if I wasn't there. Sometimes it would settle a bit during the day, but he was still gasping for air. The following Monday was the 18th December and I had arranged with my mum and Vanessa to go Christmas shopping for mum's gift. It's a bit of tradition for the two of us to take mum to pick out her present, so the day before I asked Paul if he would mind if I went. He told me to go ahead as long as Lee and Adam were with him and I had my mobile phone with me. I was nervous – this would be the first time that we were apart since he had come out of the hospital, but I was looking forward to spending some time out and about.

During the day Paul was quite breathless and he began to go a pale-greyish colour. He got a bit panicky as the time came for me to leave and asked me not to go. But I couldn't disappoint my mum and sister at such short notice. Besides, I thought that he was just getting nervous because I was leaving and maybe it would do him good to realise that he could be without me for a bit. I told him I would hurry back and that, if he didn't feel better by the time I returned, we would go to casualty. I kissed him and turned up his oxygen before I left.

After we finished buying presents, we went to the supermarket. I called home and Adam assured me that Paul was

Coming home

alright, so Vanessa, mum and I carried on shopping. By now a couple of hours had passed, so I decided to call again, because we were thinking of having a cup of tea in the supermarket café before heading home. This time, Adam told me that Paul was having some difficulty breathing, but that he would be fine until I got back. We had tea, but I wasn't very good company, so we didn't stay very long. I dropped my mum and sister at their homes and then rushed home to Paul. When I got there, Paul looked quite a bit worse than when I had left just a few hours ago. Perhaps he had been frightened without me. He just sat in his wheelchair, gasping and looking at the floor. He was very grey. Once I arrived, Adam and Lee went upstairs. It was hard for them to see their father like this. I put my arm around him and told him that we would have to call for an ambulance. "No," he said, alarmed at the idea of having to go back to the hospital. "Give it an hour or so and let's see if it settles now that you're home."

I agreed, but we both knew that it was pointless. I made tea and tried to get him to relax, but he couldn't even speak for lack of breath. Paul was slowly suffocating, so I called an ambulance and it came within ten minutes. As soon as they saw him, the ambulance men said that Paul would have to go back to the hospital, so I shouted up to Adam and Lee that we were going off and we left.

Chapter 8

Back to hospital

Paul was taken into resuscitation when we arrived at the hospital. The doctors were quite worried as his sats (oxygen saturation in the blood) was very low. The junior doctor who took charge of him had treated Paul the last time he was in the hospital. At first I was told by one of the nurses that I would have to wait outside while they worked on Paul. I protested, but didn't want to cause any trouble and was afraid I would just prevent them from seeing to Paul if I made a fuss. It wasn't long until the junior doctor came out and asked me if I could come in and help them calm Paul down. I rushed in and found Paul sitting up in bed with an oxygen mask on. His colour had gone very grey now. The doctor apologised to me for having been made to wait outside and asked me to describe what was wrong with Paul. She asked me what medications he was on and what his symptoms had been before he was brought in to the hospital. She was worried that Paul's breathing might stop altogether, so she contacted the doctor in the ITU. She was told that he was busy in maternity doing an emergency caesarean and we would have to wait before he could come down to see us. So we waited.

By now, Paul was not responding to anyone and couldn't even acknowledge me. Sometimes I could barely see him breathe. I was terrified, so God only knows how he felt. The junior doctor had administered medication to help Paul relax, thinking that would help ease his breathing. It did improve over the next hour, but only slightly. Finally the doctor from the ITU arrived from the maternity ward. He took one look at Paul and decided that he needed to be admitted to the ITU for a tracheotomy. Paul's windpipe was closing because of the stridor – the scar tissue from being ventilated when he had gone into a coma after being discharged in renal failure in September – and he wasn't getting enough oxygen into his lungs. At the time, there were no beds available in the ITU, so the doctors talked about taking Paul over to the hospital in Sheffield, where there was apparently room.

At this point they went outside the room to confer. I began to get nervous, because I thought it must be something fairly serious if they didn't want me to hear it. I could hear them anyway, as they weren't far away and they were saying that they didn't want to transfer Paul to another hospital. I wondered why. A call came through just then from the ITU that settled the matter. There was a patient who could be moved out the next day, so if the emergency assessment unit could handle Paul overnight, they would take him first thing in the morning. I asked if I could stay with Paul and the junior doctor said they would be happy for me to do that. So I just sat and held his hand that night. It was strange how I still felt safe in the hospital, despite all that they had done to Paul. Perhaps it was just that I was scared of being on my own with him and felt I wouldn't know what to do if he started to get really ill. I suppose I still believed in the training of the medical staff, even though they had disappointed me on so many occasions.

Paul was doing a bit better the following morning. He had an oxygen tube inserted into his nose and, though he was still gasping, it was a lot less severe. In the middle of the morning, a new physiotherapist came to see Paul. He needed to do work on Paul's chest to bring up all the secretions and make sure his lungs stayed clear. He explained to me that we all have these secretions, but healthy people will bring them up their windpipes throughout the day and then swallow them. Someone like Paul, who had difficulty in breathing, couldn't bring them up, which could then cause chest infections and pneumonia. Normally what would happen is that the physio would manipulate the patient's chest a bit, then put a suction tube down their throat. The tube would make them choke the secretions up and then they would be suctioned off into a little tub. However, when the physio tried to put the tube down Paul's throat, it wouldn't go. Eventually he gave up and had to leave.

Back to hospital

Later that day, Paul was moved back to the ITU, where his breathing continued to worsen. An X-ray was done, which showed that Paul did indeed have pneumonia in his right lung. A course of antibiotics was started for that. Paul didn't want me to go home that night, but I told him that I needed to get some rest if I was going to be of any use to him the next day. I tried to reassure him that he was safe now that he was back in the ITU and promised to be back at 7:30 in the morning to see him. He finally agreed and it was about midnight when I headed home. I hugged and kissed him and told him that I loved him. I couldn't look at him as I left. I had tears in my eyes and I was sure he did too. It was heartbreaking seeing him in a hospital bed again, and so soon. I cried and cried that night in bed, alone again. Every time I thought I couldn't cry any more, I would find more tears. I never would have thought it was possible for anyone to cry for anyone as much as I did for Paul that night.

The next day, I started my hospital routine again: getting up at 6.00 am to shower, then calling the hospital around 7.00 to see how Paul had spent his night, before rushing over there to see him. Sometimes the doors to the ITU would still be locked when I got there and I would have to wait for the nurse to let me in. Everyone had to wash their hands when coming into the ITU to reduce the risk of infection. As I washed, I could see Paul and it was lovely to see his face light up at the sight of me.

Christmas was only five days away and it seemed so strange to be spending the time here, instead of shopping for a turkey and presents or at home decorating the tree. Christmas was the best time of year for us as a family; we were all like little children when it came to this holiday. I was told that as long as Paul's pneumonia was under control, there was no reason that he couldn't be home for Christmas. I was determined for that to happen and I knew that even if it wouldn't be quite as it had been every other year, I would do my best to make it a happy one.

Paul's breathing deteriorated again that morning, so they put a horrible mask on him that completely covered his face. It was linked to a ventilator and forced him to breathe by pumping air into the mask, so that it had nowhere to go but down into his lungs. The nurse warned us that not many people could stand it for long, as it made them feel very claustrophobic. She told Paul to keep it on as long as he could and he managed to last about ninety minutes before begging them to take it off. A doctor came over to us while he was doing his rounds later that day. He looked very concerned at the state of Paul's breathing. He had one of the junior doctors phone Paul's ENT doctor and then spoke to him himself, urging him to come and see Paul. But he was told that it wouldn't be possible until the next day. He wasn't happy with that answer, so asked us if we minded him getting Paul another consultant whom he knew. Of course we were glad to be able to see an ENT doctor at all and were willing to do anything if it might help Paul's breathing.

The ENT specialist arrived just before dinner time. He was in his mid-thirties and a Coventry lad just like Paul. He examined Paul, then asked for a fibre optic camera so he could see into Paul's throat. This was the first time he had been to this hospital, but he asked a nurse to tell some of the junior doctors that they could come over and have a look if they wanted to. Several of them did. He got the camera up Paul's nose and then down into his throat, pointing things out to the junior doctors as he looked around. I didn't understand most of what he was saying to them. At the end of the examination, he came to the foot of Paul's bed where I was standing and said, "I have to operate straight away. I'm going to have to do a tracheotomy - put some tubing into Paul's throat so that he can breathe. The scarring in the throat from the ventilator is closing Paul's windpipe and I don't think he can carry on breathing too much longer on his own." Paul and I were both shocked, as we had been told repeatedly that the stridor would heal and we would have nothing to worry about. But I could see in Paul's eyes that he was willing to do anything that would help him breathe. Obviously we didn't have a choice.

I started to ask the doctor questions, wanting to find out as much about the procedure as I could, so there wouldn't be any unpleasant surprises afterwards. "How long will it have to stay there?" I began. "Will he be able to talk afterwards?"

Back to hospital

"I can't tell you exactly how long it will have to be in there," he said, "it depends on how long it takes for the scarring to settle down. I have to warn you that it might not heal properly at all. But assuming that it does heal and we can remove the tube, it shouldn't affect his voice at all."

The doctor went back to have another look at Paul's throat and noticed that one of the vocal cords had also been damaged. He spoke to the hospital staff and told them that he urgently needed a theatre in which to work on Paul. Unfortunately, they said, there wouldn't be one available until after lunch. It had been snowing heavily throughout the night and some of the staff had not been able to make it into work yet. The doctor agreed to wait, saying that he would have some food in the meantime and hope that the rest of the theatre staff arrived by then. Paul and I were both very confused about what was going on, but Paul just knew that he wanted to be able to breathe again and would do anything to make that happen. It's hard to describe how frightening it is to be in a situation where you are physically unable to take in enough air and to be faced with the possibility that your next breath might literally be your last. Paul had withstood a lot, but the thought of dying of suffocation frightened him more than anything else.

The doctor came back after his lunch to have another look at Paul. "We need to move as soon as possible," he said, "the theatre is ready now." I kissed Paul and told him I loved him and then they were wheeling my husband off again. 'Hurry back, Paul,' I thought, trying really hard not to cry this time. It must have been around 2.00 pm that Paul went in for the tracheotomy on December 20th. I spent that afternoon walking up and down the corridors of the ITU, looking over at the theatre doors every few seconds. At about 6.00 pm, Vanessa and Steve came to visit and I couldn't have been happier to see them. I needed someone to talk to, just to distract me for a few minutes.

Finally the theatre doors opened and they pushed Paul back in. Vanessa and Steve went and sat outside to give us a little bit of privacy as they brought him back to his bed space. Paul looked at me with pleading eyes, his face was tired and scared. His head was bloated and red and there was a long tube coming out of his throat.

Back to hospital

Obviously he couldn't speak, but he indicated that he was in tremendous pain and they gave him some morphine. The good thing was that he could breathe.

After a little while, one of the doctors came over to check on Paul. He looked at me and said, "in all my forty three years in the medical profession, I have never seen anything so barbaric." Then he walked away. I wasn't sure if he was referring to the tracheotomy or Paul's treatment in the hospital in general. Either way, it made me feel very uncomfortable and frightened. Later, I found out that Paul's tracheotomy had to be done without any anaesthetic at all. He had to remain awake and in the sitting position to be able to breathe, as lying down would cut off his air. Because they had done the operation so late, he could have stopped breathing at any moment. This meant that he could actually see what they were doing to him. He watched as they cut his throat open and then the surgeon had to put his fingers right into Paul's airway to get the tube in. Paul was petrified and started having nightmares after that surgery. Two doctors had to hold Paul down, one on each side, while the surgeon cut Paul's throat open and forced the tube into his airway with his hands.

Then the surgeon came out to tell me that everything had gone well. He told me that he had put in a temporary tube and that he would be back after Christmas to change it to a proper one. He also said that Paul should be able to speak again within a few days and that I should ask the hospital to contact him if there were any complications. I thanked him and wished him a happy holiday.

Steve and Vanessa came in then to see how he was doing, but could tell that he wasn't really up for company. Paul was in a lot of pain, so they simply wished him well, told him they would be back to see him again very soon and then left. I stayed with Paul through the night, just watching him and holding his hand. He did sleep a bit, but was afraid to move too much. The cut across his throat was bigger than I had thought it would be, almost three inches across. I was glad that he could breathe now, but horrified at what had been necessary to achieve it. I knew he was scared, so I stayed awake all night. That way, every time he opened his eyes, he would see me smiling at him.

94

Chapter 9

Making the best of Christmas

Christmas was fast approaching and I had to admit to myself that this might very well be our last together as a family. The thought filled me with sadness and I dreaded the possibility that Paul and I would have to spend it in the ITU. We all really looked forward to the holidays and I couldn't help but think back to the wonderful times we had had in the past. For us, Christmas had usually started at the end of November. Paul would buy onions in the supermarket for pickling – his always tasted so much better than the ones in the jars. He loved to do it, adding different ingredients to each jar to give them different flavours. He would sit there crying his eyes out as he peeled onions, wondering whether people would notice all the special things he added. Over the years he tried many things to keep his eyes from watering as he chopped the onions, but none of them were successful. It used to make me laugh to see my big, manly husband with tears running down his face as he sat in the kitchen cutting vegetables. Another of his Christmas rituals was to make homemade stuffing for the turkey. He used his mother's secret recipe and would put batches into lots of different foil containers so that we could have it all through the holidays, each one with a different flavour. On Christmas Eve we would have the stuffing with apple added, on Christmas Day there would be sausage in it and for New Year it was something else again.

I would have an open house on Christmas Eve, with family and friends free to drop in whenever they had a chance. We were all busy running around doing our last minute shopping and getting the fresh fruits and veggies in for our dinners, but it was lovely to

Making the best of Christmas

have people popping in and out all day long for roast pork and stuffing. The house smelled heavenly for days around the holidays. I would have a quick chat with whoever happened by about the presents we had bought or that we hoped others had bought for us. It was often the perfect opportunity to see people who I knew I wouldn't get a chance to see on Christmas itself.

In the evening, Paul would go over to the Coach and Horses pub where his mother worked. The 24th was also her birthday, so it was an extra special day for them. Paul would see lots of his friends there as well, all of his old school mates and such, and they would sit around laughing and talking over a few pints. He would come home about midnight and would tell me all that he had been doing and any good jokes that had been told. We would then begin arranging the Christmas presents under the tree, which was loaded down with fairy lights and tinsel. We would make four big piles, one for each of us in the house. Somehow Adam's and Lee's stacks were always bigger than ours – we almost always managed to get them what they wanted.

Adam and Lee were like little children around this time of year, no matter how old they got. Even after they stopped believing in Santa Claus, they still wanted Christmas to go the same way. Paul and I might have replaced Santa, but what happened remained the same. They would have no idea what we had bought them until Christmas morning when they opened their gifts. We had told them, when they were little, that their presents would disappear if they went downstairs without us, so on Christmas morning we would always hear them giggling and play-fighting on the landing as they waited for us. As they got older, they no longer believed in fairy tales, so we just threatened to take away their presents if they didn't wait for us. They never once went downstairs before us, but we did often hear things like, "hurry up mum! How long does it take you to brush your teeth?" Eventually, Paul and I would get tired of making them wait and couldn't wait any longer ourselves to see their faces as they opened their presents. We would come out to the landing, pretending that we weren't just as excited as they were and mumbling, "ok, ok, ok, let's go then."

Making the best of Christmas

They would tear into their gifts and, even if money was tight some years, I don't remember them ever showing any signs of disappointment. Even when they were very young, I think it was the spirit of the occasion they enjoyed, just as much as whatever presents they received. I loved the sight of the lounge carpet covered with Christmas wrapping-paper afterwards and the smell of bacon frying up for our sandwiches. After clearing away all the rubbish, we would eat breakfast and then begin cooking again for dinner.

Paul would normally leave mid-morning to collect his mother, who spent every Christmas with us. Margaret's favourite dessert was trifle and I tried every year without fail to make it. And every year without fail I got it wrong. It never set properly and I always ended up pouring it into the dishes. I never gave up though. Why I didn't just buy it at the supermarket is beyond me. Adam loved helping to cook the dinner and I would let him check on the turkey and stir some vegetables or whatever other little tasks I could think of. He would even help set the table on this special day. Lee's favourite task was to get the wine glasses out and put them around the table. We only ever had pop in them, but it did look very festive. He would also put the crackers out and later on would help carry the food to the table. None of my men were so eager to help clear the table after we had eaten the feast, but as it was Christmas they would all pitch in.

At around 4.00 pm, we would pack up lots of food for Margaret to take home and Paul would drop her off so that we could get ready to go to my parents. The boys always looked forward to this because they got to show off their new clothes and see their cousins, Jamie and Leanne. They had all grown up together and were more like brothers and sisters than cousins.

We would get to my parents around six and my mum always did a gorgeous Christmas supper. Then we played cards and games until the early hours of the morning. When the children got older, they would stay up with us, but when they were really little, we would put them to bed at my mum's so that we could carry on chatting for a bit longer. When it came time to leave, at about 1.00 am, we would wrap them all up in their coats and carry them out in the freezing cold to the car, trying hard not to wake them.

There were four days left until Christmas now and I hadn't even done my shopping. There would be no pickled onions and no homemade stuffing this year. As I thought about all that we would miss out on, I could feel the tears building up and a lump forming in my throat, but I refused to cry. I would just do my best to get as close to that as I could. I asked one of the doctors if there was any chance that Paul would be home for Christmas. "There is a slight chance," he said, "but we will have to see nearer the time. If we did let him home for the day, it would have to be with a nurse, as specialist training is needed to care for him in his condition." He looked at me a bit uncertainly and I wondered how slight this chance was. Still, if there was any chance at all, then I would work towards it.

That very day, I started learning how to care for Paul on my own in the ITU. They taught me how to suction him and how to change the dressings around the tube in his throat. I didn't really like doing it, because I felt his life was in my hands and I didn't have the confidence that a trained nurse would have. But I knew I had to learn, because Paul would not want to stay in the hospital over Christmas and would feel bad if the rest of us had to spend it there with him. The sort of daily care and looking after that his tracky required involved changing the dressing and the collar and washing around the hole in Paul's throat. I would also apply whatever creams were needed, usually a lubricant and in those early days an antibiotic as well. Also the dressing on his stumps needed to be changed every day, especially as there had been some cases of MRSA at the hospital. All of this took quite a bit of time, but it's not as though we had anything else to do while we were there and the routine helped to make both of us feel a bit more settled.

December 23rd arrived and they still had not made a decision as to whether or not they would let Paul home for Christmas Day. A doctor had given me a portable suction machine and taught me how to use it. It was quite handy as you could take it in the car with you when you were out and about. It could be charged up, so that it didn't have to be plugged in for me to use it. So if Paul had difficulties while in the car, I would be able to just pull over and take care of him. They had even found a theatre suction machine for us to take home, which was bigger and more powerful. I had done hours of training, but we could tell that some of the nurses still thought it would be risky for me to be totally in charge of Paul over Christmas.

I went out that day to do some last-minute shopping in the town. As I thought about the situation, I realised that I would have to make my own decisions, since the hospital wasn't making any. My head felt as if it was going to explode from all the pressure and stress. But I thought that if I eliminated some of the uncertainty, then maybe I could get around to planning as good a Christmas for my family as was possible. So I formulated my plans then went back to the hospital to discuss everything with Paul. As I had hoped, he agreed with me, so I then went to inform the sister on duty that we had decided Paul should remain in hospital on Christmas Day. It was a difficult decision to make for my family, but Paul and I both knew that he would be safer in the hospital. I called Vanessa to ask her if she could have my boys over for Christmas dinner. She said yes straight away and I knew she would do her best to make it special for them. Later that day I sat Adam and Lee down and explained our plans.

"I'm really sorry, boys," I began, trying to control my unhappiness at the thought that they wouldn't even have a proper Christmas to look forward to. "You know that your father has been through a lot recently and all in all we just don't think that it would be safe for him to come home for Christmas. I wish that I could be home with you, but I don't want him to be alone and I think it would be best if I spent Christmas in the hospital with him." I looked at both their faces and to my relief, even though I saw sadness, I did not see any blame. They both agreed that it was for the best, so I went on, lightening my tone and trying to put what they would have in the best possible light. "Your aunt Vanessa is very happy to have you over at hers for dinner and you'll get to spend time with your cousins. Plus, you can come in to the hospital beforehand to spend some time with me and your dad and we'll open all our presents together." I had to bite my tongue to keep from saying "just like old times." We all knew it would be nothing like old times. "I won't have much time to cook anything," I went on, "but I'll buy lots of nice stuff and we'll have ourselves a little feast. At least no one will have to drink my trifle this year," I said, in an attempt to get smiles out of them.

I wanted Paul to experience as much of the holiday cheer as possible, so on Christmas Eve I brought in all of the presents that I had bought for Adam and Lee so that he could watch me wrap them. With neither of us working, there wasn't as much to wrap as there had been other years, but I had done the best I could. After what we had all been through, we needed a bit of a treat. I made a sack for each of them and was beginning to feel more in control of the situation. I wished that I could leave them at the hospital so that Paul could see them all around him and feel as if it was Christmas, but they don't have enough space for that in the ITU – they've barely got room for all of the medical equipment that they need to properly care for their patients. We spent the whole of Christmas Eve together listening to Christmas carols on the television and holding hands. He still couldn't speak, but with notes and gestures he let me know that he couldn't wait until his voice came back, because he had a lot to tell me about what he had experienced while they were doing the tracheotomy. There were some tears shed that day, but also a lot of smiles. Paul had some visitors from his side of the family that day. The visits cheered him up, but people didn't stay very long. I think they were a bit unsettled by all that had happened to Paul.

Paul was getting used to the tracky now and feeling a bit more confident about it. I suppose at first he must have been worried that it would fall out if he moved too much, or maybe that it would be pulled out of position and he wouldn't get enough air. But now he was getting comfortable having it in his throat and had even begun to eat a little. I stayed until about midnight. I felt awful

Making the best of Christmas

leaving that night – Paul and I had never been separated on Christmas Eve since we had known each other. He tried to be brave and gave me a beautiful smile as I was leaving, but I could see the pain and fright in it. "See you bright and early in the morning," I said to him as I left. "Can't wait," he mouthed back.

On Christmas Day, I woke up at 5:30 am, showered and put on my best clothes. I loaded all of the presents for Paul, Adam and Lee into the car and then gave Sheba hers. She seemed to be coping quite well with the situation; she was content as long as she could smell Paul's clothes every night when I came home. I sat down with a cup of tea and I have to admit that I did cry a little at how much our lives had changed since the previous Christmas. Instead of Paul and I waking up Adam and Lee to open their presents, I was on my way to the hospital to see my husband and our boys would open their gifts there later. But I felt confident in us as a family and knew that we would get through it and even enjoy it. With that thought, I managed to stop my tears before they became a flood – after all, Paul would be able to tell I had been crying if I carried on much longer and then he would think he had ruined Christmas and feel sad. I wanted to get to the hospital at 7.00 am, so that I would be the first person Paul saw when he woke up. Many of the other patients in the ITU were in comas and I didn't want him seeing that first thing Christmas morning. After my tea, I gave Sheba a hug and set off.

The main hospital car park was empty of all but maybe ten cars and I felt incredibly lonely lifting the bags full of presents out of the boot. I had to carry them up one at a time, but when I got there with the first load and saw the look on Paul's face, it all felt worthwhile. I hugged him and said, "happy Christmas Paul, I love you!" It occurred to me then that I should be grateful – a month or two ago, I hadn't even known if we would get another Christmas together. So even if we had to spend it in the hospital, at least we were spending it together.

First I got him his breakfast. Food wasn't supplied in the ITU, as most of the patients were either in comas or were on tubes, which were inserted through their noses and supplied their nutrients. Either the ward next door would supply food for patients like Paul or their families would bring it in. Normally I would go down to the staff restaurant and get Paul whatever he felt like having that day. After breakfast, I helped him to bathe. There was no bathroom in the ITU. Bathing was accomplished by means of a big bowl filled with water and a flannel. Next I went on to change the dressings on his tracheotomy and stumps. He was still attached to a few tubes and his stumps hadn't yet healed, so it was a bit tricky getting him into clothes. We just about managed a pair of loose shorts and a button-down shirt. By now it was nearing nine o'clock and I was eager to give him his presents. I had bought him a sports sweat top that he wanted, as well as some aftershave and an assortment of other little bits and bobs that I was in the habit of getting him every year. He loved opening his presents and I had made sure that he had plenty to keep him busy.

While he was occupied with that, the phone rang several times. It was the family of the man in the bed next to Paul's. He was in a coma. His family wanted the nurses to wish him a happy Christmas from them, so whenever one of them would call, one of the nurses would go over and whisper their names in his ear, along with "happy Christmas". Paul and I thought it was lovely and hoped that the man could hear it on some level.

A little while later, Adam and Lee arrived carrying presents for both of us. Our eyes lit up at the sight of them – we were so proud of them for coping the way they had. Over the course of a few months, they had watched their father go from a strong, healthy man to one who couldn't walk, talk or breathe for himself anymore. But they never took this out on anyone or got angry at others. They were always respectful to doctors and nurses and always tried to understand why their mum had to be away from 7.00 every morning. In addition, they were doing very well at their jobs. They had both gone into construction, with Adam specialising in laying floors and Lee in tiling walls. Both were stable jobs and ones that they seemed to enjoy. But it was tiring work for them and I know how much Paul appreciated that they still made the time to come and see him every day after work.

Making the best of Christmas

Paul wanted to watch the boys open their presents and while they were doing that, Vanessa, Steve, Jamie and Leanne arrived. I thought it was lovely of them to come to the hospital on Christmas Day and they stayed for an hour or so. Paul and I opened our presents after the kids did. At about 1.00 pm the boys left to go to Vanessa's and the nurses brought in a little table for us. They laid it with a Christmas cloth and put out crackers for the two of us. After that, came the dinner which was beautiful. There was Christmas pudding and custard as well. Paul had both helpings since I don't really like either. The nurses had invited the boys to join us for tea in the ITU, so later on they laid the table out again and arranged a lovely little buffet for the four of us. There were trifles and sausage rolls, sandwiches and pickles and they even put music on for us. They had decorated the table nicely and there was a small TV by the side of the bed so that we could watch all the Christmas programmes. By the time Adam and Lee arrived the scene was quite cheerful, all things considered.

At the time, there were two other patients in the ITU, both of whom were in comas. One of the men had come in for an operation of some sort, which obviously had not gone well and he had ended up on life support. For a while they were not sure whether or not he would make it and I remember watching him go into what I can only assume was cardiac arrest one day shortly before Christmas. One of the physiotherapists had been working on him, trying to get the secretions out of his chest. He was being very forceful and all of a sudden all sorts of buzzers went off around the man and doctors came rushing in. They were quite cross with the physio. Even though they closed the curtain, when they realised that I was watching, I could still hear them telling him off. This little episode made me see even more clearly how fragile a hold on life the patients in the ITU had. The man survived that time, but remained in a coma throughout Christmas.

As the day went on, Paul kept nagging me about going over to Vanessa's house to enjoy myself a little with the family. I couldn't imagine myself having fun while he was lying in hospital, but I did really want to see everyone. I had the idea in my mind to head over there at around 10:30 pm just to spend a few minutes with the boys and the rest of the family. But I didn't make firm plans. I just told Paul that we would see how things went later on. By now Paul's breathing was fairly settled and the pain had decreased a bit so that he didn't need as much morphine. Still, I could tell that he was scared about something, but I couldn't quite put my finger on what. I didn't really want to ask him about it, because I was afraid that would make him think about it more and ruin the mood for himself and everyone else. I just assumed that he was frustrated at not being able to speak and that he would get over it in a few days' time when he got his voice back.

When we had finished eating, the nurses cleared away the teatime things and we watched the television for a while. We heard a bell go off, which meant that someone was at the outside door of the ITU, waiting to come in. The doors were kept locked, as they didn't want everyone just walking in and out. Seventeen people came trudging in, all of them family members. My eyes filled with tears at the surprise, I was so pleased that they had all cared enough to come and share our Christmas with us at the hospital. The kids were all there too and I knew that Paul was over the moon to see all his nephews and nieces. They only stayed for about an hour and a half, because Paul began to look strained after that, but it was a wonderful surprise for both of us.

After they left, I got Paul ready for bed. This was a major task because we had to hoist him out of bed and onto the commode. I cleaned his tracheotomy tube and waited until he was asleep before kissing him and leaving for the night. I went over to Vanessa's and, though it felt very strange to be without my husband, I was glad to see everyone. I stayed until everyone else went home, then took the boys back to our house. I called to make sure that Paul was still asleep and then went straight to bed. To be honest, though I had managed to enjoy myself, I was glad that the day was over and relieved that all had gone so well. I went to sleep happy at the thought that Paul would soon recover and get his voice back.

Making the best of Christmas

The 27th December was the day that the surgeon had said he would come back to change the temporary tracheotomy tube to a more permanent one. Once this was done, Paul would almost definitely be able to speak. Paul was a little worried, but mainly excited. For a fun-loving person who enjoyed telling jokes as much as he did, it was torture not being able to speak. One of the things that had attracted me to Paul when we first met was the way he could make people laugh. The past week had almost destroyed Paul. He could communicate with me easily enough – when you have been together as long as we have, you know what the other person is going to say most of the time anyway. He would only have to mime a word or two for me to understand what he meant. But it didn't work that way with others, who were afraid that they wouldn't understand him and would have to ask him to repeat things over and over. So they had taken to speaking to me when they wanted to ask or tell him something. He was being bypassed and was very frustrated by this. He told me that he felt inconsequential, as if he wasn't even a person anymore. I tried to reassure him by telling him that it was only temporary and would end as soon as he got his voice back. Still, I can imagine how awful it must have been for him.

When the surgeon arrived, he decided to take Paul into theatre to change the tube, in order to minimise the risk of infection. I watched as they wheeled his bed off again for what seemed like the twentieth time. I was a bit nervous, but kept reminding myself that it was just a routine procedure and that nothing would go wrong. About an hour later, Paul was brought back to the ITU. He smiled at me to show that he was OK, but he still couldn't speak. He was trying, but nothing was coming out. In the meantime, the nurse showed me how to change his new dressings.

There was no suction attached now, only the tube going into his throat. There was something called a lyofoam around the tube, between it and his skin. It was like a piece of sponge and it was there to absorb any secretions that came up from the sides of the tube. There was also a collar to hold the tube in place. I had to use sterile gloves to change the foam and collar every so often.

After about an hour or so, Paul still couldn't speak, so we asked the nurse if he could try with what they called a 'speaking valve'. Its purpose is to block off the air from coming out of the tracky tube and force it up the windpipe through the vocal cords so patients could speak again. She had to go off and get the doctor's approval first and when that was done, she brought him one. She attached it to the end of his tracky tube and I got ready to hear Paul make his first few sounds. He tried to say a few words, but within seconds felt that he was suffocating and had to take the valve off. We called the doctor over to find out what the problem was, nervous that perhaps Paul's throat wasn't healing as it should. One of the staff doctors came to take a look and quickly discovered that though Paul could take air into his throat, it had nowhere to go once it came out - the ventilator damage was so severe that his throat had completely closed tight at two points. This meant that as soon as the nurse inserted the speaking valve onto the end of the tracky tube, Paul couldn't breathe at all, so we had to take the valve off. The doctor recommended that we just give it a bit more time, saying that maybe Paul needed a little longer to get used to the new tube before trying the valve. I could see in Paul's eyes how disappointed he was, because he had been so looking forward to finally being able to speak, but at least we could hope that the problem would be fixed soon.

In the meantime, we had something else to look forward to – the possibility of Paul going home for New Year's Eve. I had been told that if I felt confident about taking care of Paul's tracheotomy and the ITU staff were satisfied that I knew how to do it properly, then Paul would be able to go home in a couple of days' time. The district nurses would be informed, so that they could check up on us and give us the support we needed. It was wonderful to think that maybe we would be able to spend part of the holiday in our own home. They left the speaking valve with us and Paul tried it several more times, but with no luck. Over the next few days, I continued to work hard with the staff to learn how to suction the tube and clean it and dress it properly. I was incredibly nervous about being solely responsible for it, as Paul's life would literally be in my hands, but I knew how much he wanted to go home. I tried to reassure myself by remembering that the nurses would not let us leave if they were not confident in my ability and that the district nurses would be involved as well. Still, it wasn't easy.

The doctor came to check up on Paul and informed us that he had a stenosis. This was scarring in the windpipe caused by being ventilated. It was rare and he told us again how much he wished that, of all people, it had not happened to Paul. It should clear up in time, he said, and then Paul should get his voice back. It was the 29th December, when Paul was finally discharged. The hospital policy was that no one could be discharged straight from the ITU, so he had to be transferred to a ward first and then have his paperwork sorted out there before he could be fully discharged. It was a mild annoyance as we were so eager to get home, but with some prodding of the staff on duty, we were through in a couple of hours. I can still remember the smile on Paul's face as he got his first taste of fresh air outside the hospital doors.

Chapter 10

The cover-up

The first few days after Paul came home from the hospital were difficult for me, in terms of taking care of him. I had a lot to learn and I had to do it quickly. The hospital had only sent us home with one change of dressing, telling me that the district nurse would bring over a supply for me. But it was the holidays and of course things got delayed and no one came for five days. The dressing around the tracheotomy should have been changed every day to prevent infection, particularly if it got wet. Paul showered every day, so I had to take care not to get the collar wet for those first few days, until we got more bandages. It began to get smelly and dirty, which made me very anxious as Paul, in his weakened state, was very vulnerable to infections - even a very minor ailment could endanger the life of someone in his condition.

Eventually the district nurses began to visit and expressed their surprise and concern that the hospital had discharged Paul with only one change of dressing. They also seemed a bit worried about him not having a specialist carer on hand in case something went wrong, but worked with me to help ensure that I could take care of Paul in an emergency, at least until a medical professional got there. They had been to see us a few times before, when Paul was last out of the hospital, so they knew us fairly well. Soon they were joking with us about how nice it was that Paul had lost his voice, since he couldn't nag anybody anymore. However the loss of his voice began to seriously affect Paul, especially as it began to look like it might be permanent. He could communicate with Adam, Lee and me by mouthing the words he wanted to say – we quickly learnt to read his lips. But it was almost impossible for him to communicate what wanted to say to anyone else. He had told me long ago that he wouldn't want to live if he couldn't walk and talk and now he could do neither. He repeated those feelings to me then and I have to say that I was shocked. I would have thought that after coming so close to dying – in fact, actually dying for a few minutes – a person would want to live forever. But it wasn't me in his body, dealing with everything he had to on a daily basis. Paul had a very scared look in his eyes then and I waited, but it didn't go away. Finally I asked him what was wrong. It might seem like a stupid question when he had so much to complain about, but I wanted to know if there was something in particular that was giving him that look. He told me it was fear. He couldn't stop thinking about how the doctors had held him down to cut his throat open when they did his tracheotomy.

Paul began to notice that people were treating him differently, not speaking directly to him, but choosing to speak through me instead. He felt as though they thought he was mentally damaged. I tried to explain to him that not everyone could lip read and they were probably just embarrassed that they wouldn't understand what he was trying to say to them. Still, he would get frustrated and said he felt like a non-person. I began trying to encourage people to speak directly to him. In conversations, when people addressed questions or comments to me about Paul, I would say things like "would you like to ask Paul that? He does understand what you are saying and can respond." I said it all very politely, but still I sensed that I was embarrassing them. Those who were around us most got used to it though and Paul eventually had to accept that there would be times when people would not understand what he was trying to say and then I would have to interpret. We had arguments about it sometimes and I understood his feelings, but there was only so much I could do.

The district nurses who came to visit us sorted out the supplies that Paul would need, but it would still be a few days before they would get to us. One of them documented in our care plan that we had been discharged without adequate supplies and wrote a letter of complaint to our consultant. In the meantime, she

The cover-up

suggested that I go to the ITU at the hospital to pick up the collars and noses that we would need. The noses are small devices that are designed to act much as our own noses do. The air that goes down into our lungs needs to be filtered, but since Paul was breathing through a tube, his own nose couldn't serve the purpose, so the nose was attached to the end of the tracky. It prevented little insects and particles from going into the tube, as well as keeping in moisture so that his throat wouldn't get dry, which would lead to coughing.

I went over to the hospital to pick up what we needed and left Paul in the car. I didn't like leaving him alone, but he told me that he just couldn't go back into the ITU. I can't say that I blamed him. While I was there, I noticed a gentleman sitting up in bed, laughing and joking with his visitors. I realised that it was the same man who had been in a coma over Christmas, the one who I thought had gone into cardiac arrest when the physiotherapist was trying to get his chest clear. I looked over at him and smiled. He didn't know who I was, since he had still been in a coma when we left the hospital, but he smiled back. It was good to see him awake and doing so much better.

In addition to caring for his tracheotomy, I also had to learn how to move Paul around. He was quite a large man, so getting him in and out of the car was a major task, not to mention in and out of the house. Our front door is raised about twenty five centimetres off the pathway, so I had to tilt the wheelchair back to get the front two wheels inside and then lift the whole contraption to get the back two wheels in. To this day I don't really know how I managed it, but the one thing that Paul looked forward to every day was going out for a bit, so somehow it got done. The occupational therapist from social services told us that we could have a ramp at one of our doors, either the front or the back. The back door out to the garden had two steps, which made it more difficult to fit with a ramp. The front door, in addition to being easier to fit, provided fast access to the car, so we decided to put the ramp there, even though it meant Paul would not be able to get into our garden anymore. She arranged for someone to come and take measurements of our front door and he went off to build the ramp. Once the ramp was built, we were told that it couldn't yet be attached because slabs would have to be laid down for the wheelchair to roll off onto the ramp. However, it being winter, the weather was very damp and we had snow on the ground. The ground would have to be firm for the slabs to be laid, so it was March before the ramp actually got put on to our front door. I had been struggling to take him out every day while waiting for the ramp, so it was a huge relief when it finally arrived and I could get him out and about easily.

Paul's health began to stabilise. He had some minor complaints, but we were learning to deal with his condition. His right foot had healed perfectly, but there was a small opening on the stump of his left leg that refused to get better. It had to be cleaned every day to make sure that it didn't turn into an ulcer. We were still having difficulties with the tracheotomy, although I had become quite good at taking care of it. Some days I would have to clear it up to ten times because the secretions were so bad and, if it were allowed to fill up, Paul wouldn't be able to breathe. He couldn't do it himself because the inner tube of the tracky was very tight-fitting and his fingers were too large and not dexterous enough.

While all of this was going on, Paul became very dependent on me, following me around the house and never letting me out of his sight. Because he couldn't walk, he was afraid that if his tube did block up, he wouldn't be able to summon help in time. It was distressing to watch, particularly as he was aware of it himself. You could see the sadness in his eyes at the state that he had been reduced to. I remember one day in particular when I wanted to hoover and clean upstairs. There was no way of getting Paul up there and he was afraid to let me out of his sight, especially as I wouldn't be able to hear him with the vacuum running. He said that he would sit at the bottom of the stair and tap constantly on the banister. That way, if I heard the tapping stop, I would know to come and check on him. "Why don't you just tap if you need me?"

The cover-up

I asked, smiling at him to show him that I would do whatever he wanted if it made him feel safe. "Because if I can't breathe, I might drop off and not be able to tap for you," he mouthed, not smiling at all. I felt awful. How did our lives get to this point?

At times, I would try to convince him that the likelihood of something happening to him for the few moments that I was out of his sight was very small. Perhaps I was trying to convince myself as well. "It would only take one time and then it would be too late," he would tell me. Sometimes when I tried to make light of the situation, he would get cross with me. I remember going upstairs and crying several times, wondering whether I was being cruel to him. When I look back on it now, I know that I always did my best for him and I am sure he knew it too.

Throughout January, as Paul and I struggled to develop some sort of normal routine at home, I waited for a letter from the hospital chief executive. He had told me that he would contact me to set up a meeting sometime in January, after he had investigated our claims about Paul having been discharged in renal failure. I heard nothing, so towards the end of the month I called his office and spoke to his secretary. I explained the situation to her and she said that she would look into it and get back to me. She called me back to inform me that a meeting had been arranged at the hospital for the 13th February. Later on, we received a letter in the mail confirming the appointment.

Our appointment was for 11.00 am and both Paul and I were eager to hear what the hospital had to say. We had already had two meetings at which we got no answers, hopefully this time we would be provided with some sort of explanation. The chief executive began the meeting by inquiring about Paul's health and I brought him up to date. He then asked me which damages we thought the hospital was responsible for. I found this a bit surprising, as it was obvious to me that they were responsible for everything that Paul had gone through. But I tried to answer the question politely, listing all of Paul's various ailments – the amputations of his right foot and left leg and foot, the tracheotomy and subsequent loss of his voice and the removal of his front teeth. As the meeting went on, I began to get angry. It seemed to me that the chief executive had not looked into our case at all, despite his claims that he would do just that. I felt as if I had been in this exact position before – twice, in fact. After about forty minutes, there was a knock on the door and one of the surgeons walked in. He was the one who had told the student doctors that Paul's condition was a result of his diabetes rather than being due to dehydration and going into a coma after being discharged in renal failure. He sat down opposite me and Paul, on the same side as the chief executive. Perhaps I was just being a bit defensive, but I felt that was a clear indication of whose side he was on.

The surgeon began by asking me why I thought that something had gone wrong. I was astounded that he could look me in the face and ask me such a thing, but I tried to remain calm. I took a deep breath and answered him. "Paul's fluid balance was not monitored when he was admitted for his toe amputation," I started off, assuming I should begin at the beginning as none of them seemed to have read Paul's case file. "I had spoken to everyone concerned to make sure they knew about his water requirements beforehand. Besides that fact, a surgeon should know all of these things about his patient before he operates anyway." I was angry by now and more outspoken than I normally would be. "Paul was dehydrated twice before," I went on, "and it was definitely in his file as it had happened only three months before when he was admitted for a minor operation. It was also documented in his file from when it happened the first time. If you had looked at Paul's medical file you would have known that. Moreover, I wrote in telling management about all of this, trying to put in some kind of safety net for Paul. I got assurances from the management that he would be taken care of, but obviously this didn't happen."

By now I was furious and praying that in my anger I wouldn't start crying or say anything that would jeopardize our case. I am not a paranoid person, but I had witnessed first-hand how doctors used their education to make you feel as if you didn't

The cover-up

know what you were talking about, when in fact it was them who had made the mistake. So I took a few more deep breaths and tried to regain my calm. I had taken careful notes on Paul's condition all along the way and I wanted it to be known that the hospital had neglected him. If I got too emotional, the hospital would ignore my evidence on the grounds that I was just a hysterical wife who wasn't happy with her husband's health and was looking for someone to blame. I knew Paul would never get his leg or feet back, but at least I could do my bit to make sure that they recognised their mistake and that this didn't happen to anyone else.

At the end of my big speech, the surgeon turned to the chief executive and said, "I am not taking full responsibility for this, the nursing team are responsible too." He then went on to say to me and I believe he was being sincere, "don't you think this will live with me for the rest of my life?" The surgeon left the meeting shortly after that, wishing Paul the best. The chief executive explained to us that he would have to have a case conference with all of the consultants involved in Paul's medical treatment before he could give us any answers. He said that he would arrange that as soon as possible and we would be informed of the date. After that, he could meet with us again and would be able to explain the hospital's position. Paul and I were both disappointed at yet another delay, but since there was nothing else we could do, we agreed.

The hospital's internal meeting about Paul's case was originally scheduled for the 21st March but then postponed to the 26th since not all of the people required could make the first date. The chief executive's secretary then called us after the meeting had taken place, requesting that Paul and I have another meeting with the chief executive and the director of nursing on the 29th March. When the day of the appointment arrived, I got Paul ready, both of us feeling nervous but confident. We assumed that we would be given a fairly decent financial settlement and maybe even an apology. No amount of money could give Paul back what he had lost, but at least it would help him live out the rest of his days with proper care and as comfortably as possible.

The cover-up

This time, the chief executive's body language was quite different to what it had been during the last meeting. I had been disappointed then that he hadn't yet looked into our case, but I at least had the feeling that he was listening to us and prepared to consider what we were saying. This time he leaned back in his chair and rocked on the two back legs. Clearly the hospital had made a decision and the way he carried himself suggested to me that we weren't going to like it. I became very nervous. "We established at the case conference that Paul's fluid chart had indeed not been properly looked after," he began, but rather than being apologetic, his voice seemed confident. "Some of the charts had been done but not quite up to the standard that is expected of this hospital. But Paul was not discharged in renal failure."

I felt physically sick when I heard his words. I looked at Paul's face. He seemed as shocked as I was. How could they say that to a man who was sitting in front of them, unable to walk, unable to speak and with a tube in his throat so that he could breathe – all because of hospital neglect? Worst of all, because of the loss of his leg and feet, Paul couldn't even get up and walk out on them. He had to sit there and endure all that they were saying. I had decided that morning that it was important for Paul to attend this meeting, to hear for himself what had been decided. That was when I had thought that the hospital might offer him some kind of apology and compensation. Now I was sorry that I had brought him to hear all of this, particularly as it came from a man who kept rocking contentedly in his chair as if there was nothing at all wrong.

The chief executive then asked the director of nursing to show us the blood tests that had been done on Paul, as he was aware that I knew how to read them. She opened a folder and passed me some forms that she took out from it. They showed that Paul's creatinine level was acceptable. It was at 126 and the norm is 60-120. Slightly high, but acceptable for a hospital to discharge a patient. As I was studying the forms, I noticed the director of nursing wiping her eyes. This was not the first time she had done that in meetings with us. The chief executive, on the other hand, only seemed interested in moving the meeting along. He said that he realised that Paul's fluid balance had not been monitored as well as it should have been and that they were willing to make some kind of payment for that. I asked him for clarification and the director of nursing spoke up. "We at the hospital have the ability to offer patients who have not been cared for properly up to £20,000 in compensation," she said. Then the chief executive stepped in quickly with, "of course we are not offering you that amount, but we can talk about what you think you are entitled to."

I was still stunned that the hospital was denying that they had discharged Paul in renal failure, but I tried to concentrate on what they were saying. I focused my mind on the blood test forms in front of me and that's when I saw the date on them – 26th September. Paul had been discharged on the 27th, and late in the evening at that! "These blood tests are from the day before he was discharged," I said straight away. I felt my hope begin to come back. Could it be a simple mistake? Had they just not noticed the date?

"That doesn't matter," the chief executive said quickly. "The medical staff had looked at it at the time and, on the basis of the most recent chemical data, decided that Paul was not in danger of renal failure. Even though the fluid balance sheets had not been comprehensively completed, his condition was stable enough to allow them to discharge him."

"But these tests were taken on the morning of the 26th," I went on, almost pleading. "What if his condition deteriorated over the next day and a half? Which it did!" I couldn't believe that they were trying to deny responsibility. I felt the blood rushing to my face and for the first time in the meeting felt out of my depth. Here I was sitting opposite the chief executive of the hospital and the director of nursing. What did I know compared to them? If they could show the possibility that Paul was not in renal failure when he was discharged, then I would have no chance against them in the eyes of the NHS. I don't remember the exact words that the chief executive used after that, but the gist of it was quite clear. I was entitled to my own opinion, but it would not affect the outcome of the case.

"I'll go to the newspapers!" I said, willing to try anything to get a bit of justice after all that we had been through. "I'll tell them how badly Paul was cared for while at this hospital!"

"That's your choice," he replied, still seeming quite calm, "but if you choose to do that, then all communication between us will have to cease."

"We have nothing left to say to one another anyway, if you're saying that you didn't cause the damages to Paul," I answered. He and the director of nursing just looked at me. I was quite confused at this point. I had waited so long for this meeting and yet it had never occurred to me that this might be the outcome. Could I really take on the whole hospital? Even if I could, how long would it take before Paul and I saw any justice? Would we be better off cutting our losses and just trying to make the best of the rest of our lives with what little the hospital was willing to offer us? I took a minute to clear my mind. Then I decided I would try to leave my options open and in the meantime gather as much evidence as I could. So I asked them to forward me copies of the photos taken of Paul's leg and feet before they were amputated.

I wanted to get Paul out of there as soon as possible and began to wrap things up. Before I left, the chief executive asked me if I was going to be available for the first User Involvement Programme meeting set for the following week. This was a new programme that the director of nursing had spoken to me about beforehand. It was set up by the government and allowed people who had bad experiences in hospital to come in to talk about them with the staff. I had been eager to participate in this as I felt that, if it would help to keep what had happened to Paul from happening to someone else, then it was worthwhile. I said yes to his question, but at that point I really just wanted to get out of there.

Paul was very upset when we got outside, so I stopped the wheelchair and went around to the front. I leaned over and hugged him and said, "look at me Paul." He did and I don't think I had ever seen anyone look so sad. I was furious at the hospital for making him feel this way, especially after all the damage they had already inflicted on him. "I will fight for you Paul, until we get the truth."

"Yes, I know," he mimed back to me, "but will I be alive to see it?"

We drove around for an hour or so after the meeting before going home, trying to clear our heads. Paul asked me not to tell the boys the details of what had gone on. He felt ashamed and inadequate in some way, as though what had happened was his fault. He thought the boys and everyone else would think that he had caused his medical problems because he was overweight and used to smoke. I was at a loss to know what to do. So I just told Adam and Lee that the hospital was making things a bit difficult for us, but that it would be alright in the end.

When we got home, I kept playing the facts over in my mind, trying to work out if I had a strong enough case to take a stand against the NHS. I felt so small facing such a huge organisation, filled with doctors and nurses who had a lot more education than I did and who would probably be able to argue rings around me. I didn't want to discuss things with Paul or the boys, because that would only worry them further.

The next morning, I called the chief executive to tell him that I would not be able to come into the hospital that Monday as we had planned. Although I was very interested in the User Involvement Programme, under the current circumstances I didn't feel that it was a good idea to become a member of the team. I wasn't yet sure what actions I would be taking against the hospital, but since it seemed I was disputing the level of Paul's care with the administration, I didn't want to make things more difficult for myself by getting involved further with them. The chief executive told me that it was fine if I didn't want to be involved, but if I changed my mind in the future then they would love to have me on their team.

After speaking to him, I called my solicitor. All she had at this stage was the report from the first dehydration episode. I brought her up to date on Paul's medical condition. She said she would write to the hospital to get Paul's updated files and then would contact me. I was quite cross with her for letting things lapse, but I felt that my hands were tied. When you're on legal aid and not paying, then people seem to do what they want when they want.

The following day, I got a very important phone call – it was the first thing to happen that made me think that maybe we did have a chance against the NHS after all. When I answered, I heard a woman on the other end. She told me that she was a nurse at the hospital and that the administration had been lying to me. She claimed that there had been another blood test done on the 27th September and that the results were in Paul's file, as well as on the hospital computer. This test revealed that Paul's creatinines had risen from 126 to 200 – a definite indication that he was going into acute renal failure. At first I didn't believe her. Surely, after all that Paul had suffered at the hands of that hospital, they wouldn't lie to us and try to keep what little compensation he should get away from him? I didn't believe that anyone could be so cruel. She told me that she would mail me a copy of the blood test results as proof, as well as sending a copy to our GP and keeping several for herself. She also told me that she was afraid of losing her job if anyone in management ever found out that she had told us of the existence of the 27th September blood test results. So she talked about what I had to do to keep her safe and not implicate her in my case. She made me go over and over what I had to do to keep her identity hidden, so that there would be no mistakes. At this point I was willing to do whatever she said if she could give me proof of the second blood test.

After I got off the phone with her, I sat and tried to think of the best way to explain all of this to Paul. I had almost fainted when I heard the news – what would his reaction be? I was literally afraid that the shock would do him bodily harm. Stress can be very dangerous for someone in his delicate condition. I broke the news to him as gently as I could, trying to stress the positive possibilities of this news. Maybe with this new document, I suggested, the

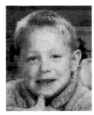

Paul, aged six.

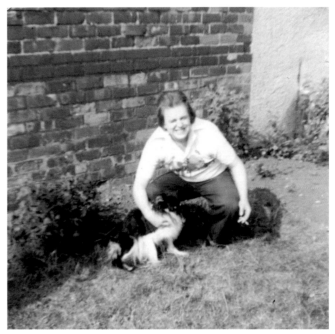

Paul aged nineteen with Cindy – a Shetland Collie I bought for Paul's dad Doug.

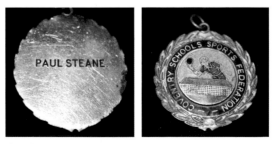

Paul loved sports – he played for a Sunday football team and won several medals for table tennis.

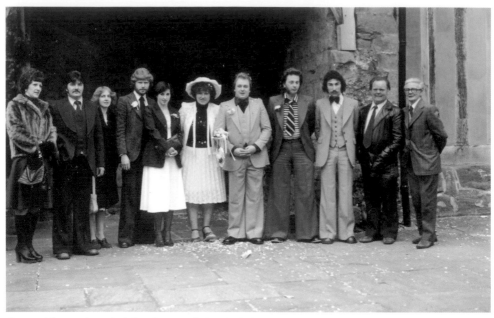

Our wedding – please don't laugh at our clothes, back then we thought these were pretty cool.

Paul, myself and the boys on holiday in Weymouth.

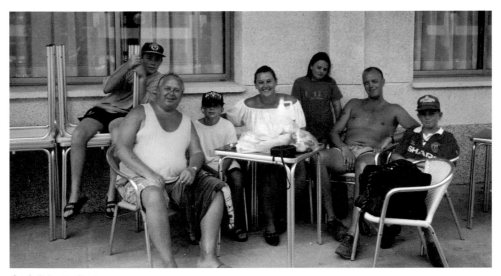

On holiday in Spain.

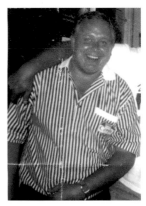

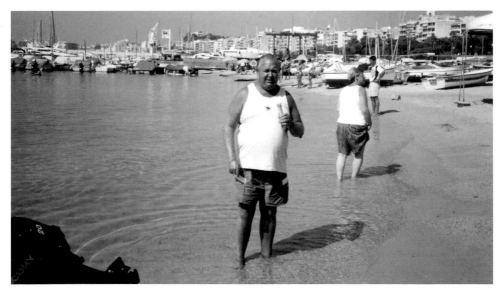

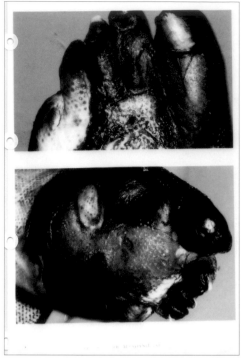

Paul's left foot before his left leg was amputated.

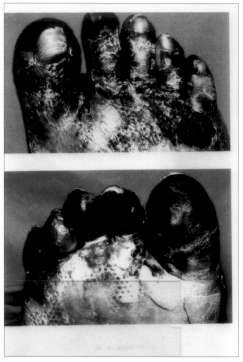

Rot on Paul's right foot before the toes and most of the foot were amputated.

"Had Paul been treated correctly while in a coma, there would have been no damage at all to his feet."

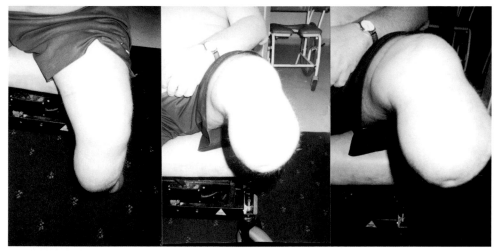

The stump of Paul's left leg – this never healed sufficiently for Paul to use his prosthetic leg.

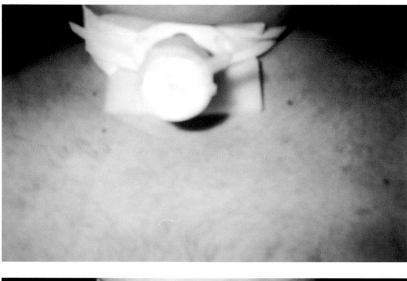

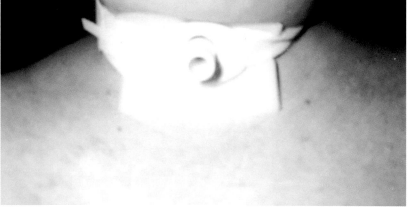

Paul's tracheotomy (tracky) – two doctors had to hold Paul down while another cut his throat to insert the tracky without an anaesthetic.

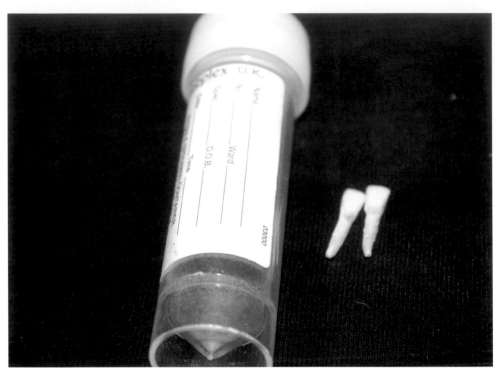

The hospital gave me a jar with Paul's two front teeth which the doctors knocked out while trying to ventilate him when he went into a coma after being discharged in renal failure.

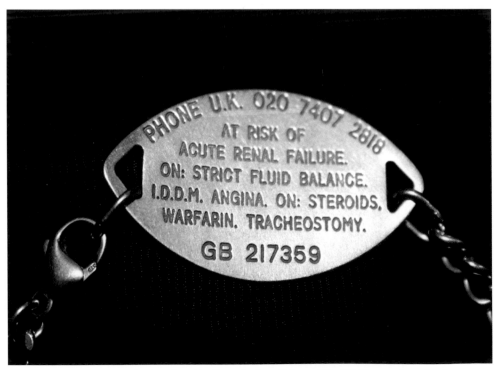

The hospital gave us a bracelet describing Paul's medical condition so if he fell ill somewhere else, doctors would know about his medical problems (caused by the hospital's negligence).

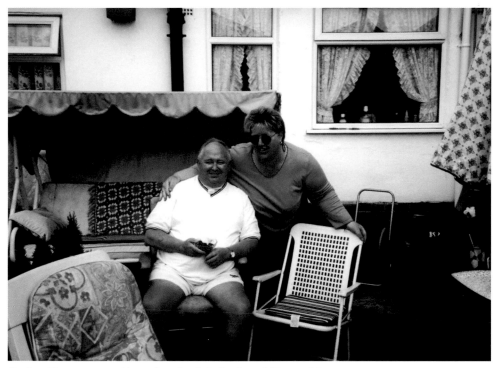

Paul and I at my parents' bungalow shortly before he took his own life.

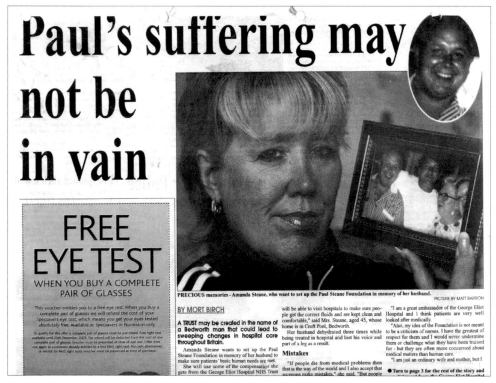

Paul's suffering may not be in vain

PRECIOUS memories - Amanda Steane, who want to set up the Paul Steane Foundation in memory of her husband.
PICTURE BY MATT BARRON

FREE EYE TEST
WHEN YOU BUY A COMPLETE PAIR OF GLASSES

This voucher entitles you to a free eye test. When you buy a complete pair of glasses we will refund the cost of your Specsavers eye test, which means you get your eyes tested absolutely free. Available at Specsavers in Nuneaton only.

To qualify for this offer a complete pair of glasses must be purchased. Free sight test available until 20th December 2003. The refund will be deducted from the cost of one complete pair of glasses. Voucher must be presented at time of eye test. Offer does not apply to customers already entitled to a free NHS sight test. No cash alternatives or refund for NHS sight tests. Voucher must be presented at time of purchase.

BY MORT BIRCH

A TRUST may be created in the name of a Bedworth man that could lead to sweeping changes in hospital care throughout Britain.

Amanda Steane wants to set up the Paul Steane Foundation in memory of her husband to make sure patients' basic human needs are met.

She will use some of the compensation she gets from the George Eliot Hospital NHS Trust will be able to visit hospitals to make sure people get the correct fluids and are kept clean and comfortable," said Mrs. Steane, aged 45, whose home is in Croft Pool, Bedworth.

Her husband dehydrated three times while being treated in hospital and lost his voice and part of a leg as a result.

Mistakes

"If people die from medical problems then that is the way of the world and I also accept that surgeons make mistakes," she said. "But people

"I am a great ambassador of the George Eliot Hospital and I think patients are very well looked after medically.

"Also, my idea of the Foundation is not meant to be a criticism of nurses. I have the greatest of respect for them and I would never undermine them or challenge what they have been trained for - but they are often more concerned about medical matters than human care.

"I am just an ordinary wife and mother, but I

● Turn to page 3 for the rest of the story

Our local newspaper was horrified at what had happened to Paul.

Dear Dr. ███████████ enclosed are photocopies of Paul Steane's blood results on the day of discharge from ███████████ Hospital. Mrs. Steane had been trying to track these down without success - I have found them in the notes, as she was told they were not on the computer at ███████████

I'm afraid these results confirm her suspicions - his Creatinine had jumped from 126 on 26/9██ to 200 the following day: Reasonable evidence that he was developing A.R.F. prior to discharge. I'm sure Mrs. Steane will find this information useful

Not To be Removed.

"Dear Dr. xxxxx - enclosed are photocopies of Paul Steane's blood results on the day of discharge from xxxxx xxxxx hospital. Mrs Steane had been trying to track these down without success - I have found them in the notes, as she was told they were not on the computer at xxxxx xxxxx.

I'm afraid these results confirm her suspicions - his creatinine had jumped from 126 on 26/9/xx to 200 the following day: reasonable evidence that he was developing A.R.F. (Acute Renal Failure ed.) prior to discharge. I'm sure Mrs. Steane will find this information useful."

A nurse, angered by the way Paul had been treated, sent me copies of the blood tests done on the day of Paul's discharge from hospital. At first, hospital management claimed the blood tests had never been done. When I told them the tests had been done, they then said the results had been 'lost'. The 'lost' blood tests proved that Paul had been going into renal failure when he was discharged from the hospital. Being discharged in renal failure led directly to Paul going into a coma and eventually losing his legs, voice and ability to breathe properly.

The cover-up

hospital would be willing to admit their fault quickly and we wouldn't have a long drawn-out battle ahead of us. But he got a sad look on his face that would be there more and more often in the next couple of years. He tried to explain to me what he was feeling, but was too emotional. Eventually he managed to get his worries out – how would he ever be safe again? If the hospital was willing to tamper with his medical files and suppress the truth, then how could he ever rely on them again? What would happen the next time he fell ill and had to be readmitted? I tried to reassure him, but what could I say? Deep down, I felt that he was right. I told him that this sort of thing wasn't normal, but how did I know that? Perhaps it happens all the time and not everyone is as lucky as we were to have someone with enough conscience to call and reveal the truth. I kept telling myself that most of the hospital staff we had met were honest and decent people. But obviously there were some who weren't,

Paul felt that he was losing what little control over his life that he had. We were both anxious now that something would happen and we would never get this second test in the mail. What if the nurse who had called us lost her nerve and decided not to send it to us after all? We couldn't wait until we had it in our hands.

After the last meeting with the hospital on the 29th March, I had asked them to send me a letter stating in writing what they had informed me of then. Within two weeks, I received a letter dated 12th April from the chief executive, which stated that the latest blood test for Paul was done on the 26th September. The chief executive claimed that this blood test showed that Paul was not in renal failure and was well enough to be discharged:

We are able to advise you that in essence the conclusion of our discussions were that the maintenance of Paul's fluid balance record was below the standard that we would expect to see and consequently gave only a partial indication of Paul's level of input and output. At our meeting the medical staff did, however, refer to a pathology report undertaken on 26th September 200X, which they

The cover-up

believed did not indicate that Paul was in renal failure upon his discharge. We, therefore, were of the view that whilst Paul's fluid balance had not been comprehensively completed, on the basis of the advise (sic) provided to us the latest chemical picture did not indicate that this had resulted in Paul's renal failure.

Just after we received this letter from chief executive denying that Paul had been in renal failure at his discharge, we got the blood test result from the 27th September that had been promised to us by the nurse who had phoned us. Along with it was a letter, which read:

Enclosed are photocopies of Paul Steane's blood results on the day of discharge from ------------ Hospital. Mrs Steane has been trying to track these down without success - I have found them in the notes, as she was told they were not on the computer at the hospital.

I'm afraid the results confirm her suspicions - Paul's creatinine levels had jumped from 126 on 26/9 to 200 the following day; reasonable evidence that he was developing A.R.F. (acute renal failure, ed.) prior to discharge. I'm sure Mrs Steane will find this information useful.

The letter was signed, but I had promised never to reveal the identity of the nurse and I never have. Also included in the envelope was a copy of Paul's discharge letter. This read, *"Effective admission for amputation of left 5th toe. Good post op recovery."* This form had also been mislaid or removed from Paul's medical files.

At the bottom of the chief executive's letter, he had added that if I needed any further assistance, I should not hesitate to call his office. He would be on holiday for two weeks, but the director of nursing would be happy to speak to me. So I phoned her. "Hello," I said when she answered, "I have copies of blood tests for Paul dated the 27th September. Could you please go to your computer and bring them up?" When she began speaking, I could

122

The cover-up

tell by her voice that she was shocked. Paul was sitting at my side, desperately trying to hear the conversation and I felt so pleased to see the satisfied look on his face.

"What do they say?" she asked me, as though she didn't already know.

"They say that Paul's creatinine levels had risen to 200 on the day of discharge," I informed her. I would have been pleased if I hadn't been so angry at what all of this had done to my husband.

"Can I look for the results on my computer and then call you straight back?" she asked me. "OK," I agreed, wondering who she would call when she got off the phone with me and what they would agree between themselves to say to us. For a moment I was surprised at myself for being so paranoid, because it wasn't like me. But after all they had done to us, I felt I had good reason to be suspicious.

It took her about thirty minutes to call us back. She said that she had found the blood test results and had taken them to one of the surgeons, who confirmed that Paul had in fact been in renal failure when he had been discharged. I told her how upset Paul and I were at what had happened and that we wanted a meeting with the chief executive as soon as possible. That evening Paul's mood was a bit lighter, which was good to see. I suppose he thought that things would be easier for us from then on. I was not so sure, but was glad to see him a bit happier. I was still very angry. I kept seeing Paul sitting in front of the chief executive and director of nursing at our last meeting, unable to walk out when they denied that he had been in renal failure, or even to tell them what he thought. I was terribly upset by everything that had gone on and I wasn't sure what to believe - that professionals entrusted with our health care could be so careless as to misplace the results of a blood test, or that someone had done it deliberately in order to hide their own mistake and cheat someone out of their well-deserved compensation. Paul could not walk or talk and had been on the brink of death. How could they not admit that he deserved some form of compensation, not to mention their deepest apologies? How dare they treat us so appallingly?

The cover-up

The following day, Paul had an appointment at the hospital with his rheumatologist. When we came out, we were told by the nurses that the director of nursing had come looking for us and that she was waiting to speak to us. When we sat down, the first thing I told her was how disgusted I was by all that had happened. I made it clear that I believed that things were being covered up, even though I couldn't begin to guess why. She told Paul and me that she had contacted the chief executive on holiday and that he wanted to meet with us that Thursday at 11.00 am. She expressed her regret and said that she was shocked that this second blood test had been 'lost'.

By this time, our GP had also received copies of the missing blood tests with the covering letter, as the nurse had said he would. Our GP said he felt let down and embarrassed by the hospital. He confirmed that Paul had been discharged in renal failure and said how sorry he was that Paul had ended up the way he had because of the hospital's neglect. Paul and I both felt a little better knowing that not every doctor was against us.

It was nearing the end of April now and I was getting more and more frustrated with our solicitor. She had been brought up to date on Paul's condition, but still had not been to see him or even asked for statements from the hospital about either incident of dehydration, despite saying that she would during our last phone conversation though at least we had the report from the kidney specialist in London after Paul's first incident of renal failure. This stated that the clinical care that Paul had received was not up to even minimum standards and that this had caused him to go into renal failure. Thinking back on this report, I found myself wondering if Paul's case was unique. If it had happened just once, I would have said that it was just a freak accident. But the fact that it had happened to the same person three times over the course of just sixteen months made me doubt its rarity. There must be more people dying in our hospitals from lack of water and they and their families aren't even aware of it.

When the day for the next meeting with the chief executive came around, Paul and I got there half an hour early, as it was

The cover-up

difficult getting the wheelchair in and out of the hospital administration building. At about five minutes to eleven the chief executive and the director of nursing came in to greet us and showed us into the chief executive's office. "How did you find out about the blood tests?" he began straight away.

"Someone called us on the phone," I said and then added quickly, "but I was asked never to reveal their identity and I won't. And I just want to say right away how disgusted we both are that the hospital tried to cover up what has happened to Paul."

This time, the chief executive's attitude towards us was a lot different than it had been at the last meeting. There was no more rocking in his chair now. He admitted to us that this was the biggest embarrassment of his career and assured us that he would find out how it had happened. He began by telling us about some faults in the hospital filing system, but his explanation went nowhere near explaining how Paul's blood test results from the 27th, the critical ones that proved that he had been discharged in full renal failure, had been "misplaced" from both his file and the hospital computer. (Much later, I found out that the chief executive must have known all the time that the last blood tests had been done on 27th September and not the 26th September as he claimed. Before our 29th March meeting with the chief executive, at which he had maintained that the last blood tests done on Paul had been on 26th September, the chief executive had requested that Paul's medical files be updated. Paul's files were fully updated by 23rd March and the blood test results from the 27th September, which proved Paul had been discharged in renal failure, had been reprinted for the chief executive on 22nd March – seven days before our 29th March meeting at which he denied there had been any blood tests done on Paul on 27th September).

The chief executive said that for now the insurers were admitting liability for the damages done to Paul and went on to assure us that the hospital would do everything to make sure things were taken care of smoothly and efficiently. I wasn't quite sure how to take all of this, as I had heard similar words from him already. Still, I thanked him and said that they were being very kind. The director of nursing then began talking about the legal side of things. She said that normally a solicitor would write and ask for a patient's notes to be prepared and that this could take weeks, but that since the hospital wanted to sort things out as soon as possible, she would get everything ready to be sent as soon as our solicitor contacted the hospital. In addition, she said, anything else that our solicitor required would be made available to her upon request. She then informed us that the insurers were willing to give us one or more interim payments, until we had the final settlement and that our solicitor would have to apply for these. This was all good news to us, obviously, but there was still the issue of the blood tests. I didn't want them to think that we would stop asking about that, just because they were now finally offering us some compensation. We still wanted a full explanation of how they had gone missing and not just some excuse about faulty filing. I explained that Paul felt very unsafe knowing that important test results could simply be taken out of his file and that we wanted an inquiry. I also voiced the possibility that this sort of thing was happening far more often than anyone cared to admit and how serious the implications of that possibility were. I wasn't sure exactly what I could do about others dying due to poor care, but I just felt I had to make it known that we weren't stupid and that we, and others, were becoming aware of the problem.

As we were leaving, the director of nursing asked me again if I would take part in the User Involvement Programme training courses that we had discussed earlier. Now that it seemed as though our disputes were coming to an end, I was more eager to do it. I told her yes and we left.

Chapter 11

Trying to rebuild our lives

Since his discharge from the hospital at the end of December, Paul had been attending amputation classes twice a week, on Tuesdays and Thursdays. The ambulance would come for him at around 8.00 or 8:30 am, so I would get him up at 7.00 to be showered and dressed on time. In the beginning, I was scared to death about letting him go anywhere without me, in case something should go wrong and I wasn't there to look after him. But I reasoned with myself and realised that he was going to a hospital, so if anything went wrong they would be able to handle it. Strange how I still thought he was safe in hospitals, even after all that had happened. He found the classes difficult at first – no one would speak to him because they found it hard to understand him when he responded. For someone as outgoing as he was, this was hard to deal with. He asked me to see if I could go with him to help communication. But the hospital refused. They told us that there wasn't room in the classes for the families of patients. Anyway, as the year went on, Paul got more comfortable there and the other members of the class began to learn how to understand him. Soon he was a very important part of the group and he loved going. He made quite a few good friends there and was causing havoc again just like his old self.

I was very happy for him that he could have this bit of life on his own, independent of me. I never found him a burden and always tried to make this clear to him, but I could see in his eyes how he felt and knew I would feel the same in his situation. When you lose a limb or the ability to do things you used to take for granted, like walking and talking, you don't feel like a whole person anymore. You begin to feel useless and completely dependent on whoever is taking care of you. For someone as feisty as Paul, this is very hard to deal with. I was glad he could get out a couple of times a week and "socialise" a bit. Not to mention that it gave me a bit of much-needed time for myself.

I imagine that an eagerly awaited moment in any amputee's life is when they are first fitted with their prosthesis. The stump of the missing limb has to be completely healed and all the swelling gone before this can be done. Normally this will take from three to six months. Every month or so, on a Friday, Paul would attend another amputation clinic at the hospital about his prosthesis. I remember that Paul couldn't wait to try on his new limb and he was very emotional the first time that he did it. There was a very tight latex sock with a bolt in the end that was meant to go under the stump and connect it to the prosthesis. It had to be rolled onto the leg, but Paul couldn't do this because of his arthritis, so I had to help him with it. Once that was in place, the leg could be screwed on and then came the moment that we had both been waiting for. Paul stood up again. His wheelchair was placed between two bars and he hoisted himself up and walked along holding on to them. I couldn't hold back my tears. My man was standing again! I hadn't seen this for over seven months. He looked over at me for encouragement and there were tears in his eyes too. His bottom lip quivered and he had to look away to hide his emotions. I wanted to run over and tell him how proud I was, but I couldn't. The hospital staff were quite strict about this. They didn't want anyone distracting him because he could so easily fall over. He was allowed to take his prosthesis home then, but told not to use it. He still had a long way to go and his physiotherapists were insistent that he not rush things and injure himself. They wanted to make sure that it was safe for him to use the leg at home.

In the meantime, I was still undergoing training at the hospital for Paul's tracheotomy. The incision in his neck was still relatively new, so Paul was afraid that when I took the tube out, the scar might close and he wouldn't be able to breathe. I used to get very anxious myself, but put on a brave face for Paul so that he wouldn't get even more nervous. At first it was difficult finding the right tube for Paul. They come in various sizes and it can be very uncomfortable for someone with a tracheotomy to have someone else trying to stick a tube into their neck that doesn't fit. This can aggravate the throat, which causes coughing. The coughing could then either bring up phlegm, which could get stuck in the tube or else the phlegm would remain in his chest and harden, thereby blocking his breathing. There was a stage where Paul was waking up every morning with hard plugs of phlegm, which he would try to cough up for a while, before giving up and going on the nebulizer. This would moisten his windpipe and make it easier to bring up whatever needed bringing up. Sometimes I would have to use suction to bring it up, which he hated because it made him feel sick. He told me a few times that if he had to have that done regularly, then he wouldn't have been able to cope. He ended up going on the nebulizer up to eight times a day, because he hated the suction so much.

He also didn't want to go out around this time, because he was embarrassed to be coughing up phlegm through a tube in front of other people. I told him that no one could really see it, as it went straight into a tissue and that anyway people didn't mind things like that when the person clearly has no other choice. I told him that no one would fault him for it or consider it bad manners or disgusting, but he had his pride and felt that others would think him dirty.

By now we had been in and out of the hospital so many times, that we had been introduced to nearly all of the management. They invited us to their quarterly general meetings and seemed genuinely interested in knowing our opinions. It was very refreshing for me and Paul, after feeling for a long time that no one was listening to us. At one of these meetings, we met the woman whose job it was to set up the User Involvement Programme training workshops for hospital employees where patients and carers could tell their stories of how they had been treated while in hospital or as outpatients. The idea was to create sensitivity and awareness in the hospital staff, so that they could

129

better help their patients. She had heard about us and wanted to hear our story in greater detail, directly from us. She sat and listened as I talked and seemed greatly disturbed by what I said. She had already rounded up quite a few people who wanted to become involved in these workshops and asked us if we would be interested. Paul was unsure about it at first, but I was excited right from the very start. I thought that it would be very therapeutic for both of us not only to tell our story, but to know that by educating the hospital staff, we were helping others not to suffer as Paul had.

Knowing that Paul had reservations, I told him that I would be happy to do the lectures on my own if he didn't want to take part. I could understand, after all that he had been through, why it might be difficult for him to have it discussed in front of strangers, or even to keep going back to the hospital where it had happened. I told him that he didn't have to make up his mind there and then, since we still had a little while to go before the first workshop. Over the course of the next few weeks, all the lay trainers were brought in to meetings to teach us what would be expected of us at the workshops. The plan was to have at least three different stories told at each and each person would get fifteen minutes to tell their stories. Afterwards there would be group discussions between the staff and the patients. The aim was for us to have our stories prepared, so that all the relevant points we wanted to make would be made within the time allotted. I wasn't sure if fifteen minutes would be enough for all I had to say, so I went home and got to work on our computer, doing research and noting down all the major points that I wanted to focus on. We had recently received the photographs of Paul's limbs before they were amputated, which I was also going to take with me. They were so horrendous, it was a wonder that we could look at them without crying. I decided that before I showed the pictures, I would warn people how awful they were, so that they would have the choice of looking away if they didn't want to see them.

We went to the first lecture the following week at about 10.00 am. The workshops were not compulsory, so it was the organiser's job to convince people to attend. She said this was difficult, as hospitals are always understaffed and the carers are

Trying to rebuild our lives

usually overworked. So most of the people who turned up for the first meeting were administrative and not the people who directly look after patients. It was a bit disappointing, but the organiser was very enthusiastic, so we just hoped that attendance at the workshops would improve. The first lay trainers to speak were a husband and wife, where the wife had been the patient. He did most of the talking and complained about the poor treatment she had received. She was left in pain a lot of the time and was afraid to complain. So she would take out her frustration on him when he came to visit and then he had to go and speak to the nurses for her. But they didn't listen to him. He had difficulty coping because he was still working and trying to take care of their two children at the same time. It all sounded so familiar to me.

Eventually, it was our turn. Paul was next to me in his wheelchair, with his tracheotomy and amputations clearly showing. I looked at the class and began. I started my story about how he was first admitted to hospital with a suspected stomach bleed. I told them how I watched him get progressively worse over the next ten days, not understanding how the doctors and nurses were not noticing this. I explained how we were embarrassed at being overweight and feared that we would be judged if we asked for more food or water. I went on to tell them how the hospital had thought his unhealthy look was due to psychological reasons and how they had only agreed to do more blood tests to "ease my mind" when I had insisted. From there I went on to summarise the London kidney specialist's report, which stated that Paul had suffered full renal failure and that it had been caused by poor clinical care, mainly lack of water. I told them about him being prescribed MST, a heroin derivative when he was next in the hospital and how the side effects of this confused me, so that I didn't notice his dehydration for the second time. Not that it should have been my responsibility to monitor such things anyway.

As I went through the story, there were certain parts where I would become very emotional and would feel my lips quiver and tears come into my eyes. Paul watched me very closely and would put his hand on my arm at those moments, just to give me a bit of support. I was so proud that even though my man was in a

Trying to rebuild our lives

wheelchair, he was still concerned for me and still trying to help me out. I saw a lot of people reaching for their hankies during my fifteen minutes. I had brought the blood test results from the 27th September and passed these around the class when I got to that part of the story, to show the state Paul had been in when he had been discharged from the hospital. When I finished telling them about his multiple cardiac arrests and coma, I passed around the photos of his foot and leg, to show them the damage that had been caused. I warned them that the images were pretty gruesome, but no one looked away. I told them all about the tracheotomy and how Paul remembered them ripping at his throat to get an airway and how he still had nightmares about it. I told them how our two sons had been affected by seeing their father become an invalid and how they had blamed me at times for letting him go back to the hospital. Once or twice someone had to leave the room because they couldn't take it anymore.

I summed up by saying, "when my husband came into hospital for the first time, he could walk and talk and breathe on his own. Now he can do none of those things. It has wrecked his life, both physically and mentally, as well as mine and that of our two sons. After the first incident of dehydration, I did everything I could to make sure that it didn't happen again, but Paul's basic needs were still neglected by hospital staff. I understand that there are staff shortages, that staff don't get paid enough, that there are not enough well-trained staff and so on. But none of that excuses, at least in my mind, not giving someone the water and other basic care they need! We've spent the last few months looking for answers, asking the hospital to tell us why all of this happened. They have not been able to do so yet, or to tell us how important documents could have simply vanished out of Paul's file. I suppose that, as frustrating to us as it is, we just have to settle for the fact that there are no good answers for what happened to my husband. So now we are just trying to make a difference. This is a tragedy that cannot happen again." I paused at this point, trying to make eye contact with as many people in the class as I could. I wanted to make sure that I had their attention and that they were all taking me seriously. When I could see that they were, I went on. "Whatever

Trying to rebuild our lives

you take away from this seminar, can we agree on one thing? This cannot happen to anyone else. Please."

Although Paul and I felt progressively more comfortable with each lecture, it was never easy to talk about what had happened. I suppose we experienced the horror of it again with each new audience. Perhaps some of them had heard a bit about us beforehand, but they wouldn't have known the details and certainly wouldn't have seen the pictures of his limbs before amputation. We could see the look in their eyes as we passed the photos around or got to certain sections of our story and we felt it again as though for the first time. After all of the lay trainers had spoken, the participants had the chance to ask us questions for about an hour or so. They almost always asked how we coped with daily life. Another question they always asked was about the punishment meted out to those responsible. As it turned out, the hospital had a 'no blame' policy in place, so as far as we knew, no one had ever been brought to account. I was never sure whether this was a good or bad policy. I don't think what happened to Paul was the result of the bad judgement of one or two specific people, but there were certainly some people who could have done things, and indeed said that they would, but then didn't. Many of them asked why we hadn't gone to the press. I wasn't sure how to answer that. I didn't think that I could tell them how the hospital chief executive had threatened to make life difficult for us if we involved the newspapers in our case.

As time went on, the classes became a great success and more and more people started asking if they could attend a lecture. We still had a problem getting nurses to come, because the sisters found it hard to spare them from their daily duties. Often, when we did have nurses attending the classes, they would get quite anxious about having to work with the people who had caused Paul so much injury. They would ask what wards these people had been on, or try to get other information about them. Of course Paul and I never disclosed any names, we would just say something like, "it could easily have been your ward." I remember one nurse who attended a lecture reporting back to management that, because of

133

hearing Paul's story, she had saved the life of one of her patients. I can't even put into words how good that made us feel.

As the year went by, Paul and I began to have financial difficulties. Paul obviously needed lots of things to deal with his new situation and I did what I had to do to get them. He also wanted to go places that we couldn't really afford, but after all he had been through, I was not about to say no to him. I was always aware of how precious Paul's life was and I never wanted him to lack anything ever again. He wanted to go out of the house every day, even if only for a ride in the car. He just couldn't sit inside all day long. He could no longer get into the back garden and missed it. He didn't want to sit in front of the house, because he said he was "damaging the view". I used to tell him off for saying things like that, but he would just laugh. I suppose deep down I understood how he felt. Even if it wasn't true, he must have imagined everyone walking by thinking of the man he used to be and feeling sorry for him as they smiled and waved and said hello.

We used to dream about what we would do when Paul's compensation was finally paid. We had the idea that we would get a bungalow and have a greenhouse in the back garden. Paul wanted to grow tomatoes and lettuce and everything else you needed to make a salad. He also wanted to have raised flower beds so that he could look after the plants from his wheelchair. It really excited us to talk about all this, but I would look in Paul's eyes and see him wondering if he would be around to enjoy our dream. If we ever did manage to buy this bungalow, it would have to be nearby because we couldn't venture too far from the hospital. We knew that we would be going to hospital often for the rest of our lives and Paul felt safer at a hospital which already knew about him and would know exactly what to do for him in an emergency. The hospital had finally begun to put in some safety nets to protect both Paul and themselves. I tried not to think about the fact that so much of this could have been avoided if they had only done this sort of thing sooner, as I had asked in my first letter to the chief executive. The first thing they did was to put an alert on the computer system so that if Paul was ever admitted in an emergency, it would immediately flag all his medical conditions and bring up the names

Trying to rebuild our lives

of all of his consultants so that the staff could call them for advice. They also decided that Paul was at risk with junior doctors, so one of his consultants should write a letter detailing his condition and this would be placed in the front of every volume of his file. That way, anyone who was attending to him would know what to do, even if they had never seen him before. They also talked about getting Paul a medic alert bracelet, which has a worldwide logo on it. He would wear it all the time and if he happened to be away from home, any hospital in the world could type the number on his bracelet into their computer and all of his medical files would be available to them. With all of these precautions, we were beginning to trust the hospital again and felt that they were finally working with us. Things were beginning to look up.

Since his coma, Paul had been having some difficulty with his left eye. The way he explained it was that there was a big black line across his field of view and he could see a bit above and a bit below it, but nothing in the middle. When you have trouble seeing out of one eye, it often affects the other one too and I would frequently see him watching TV with his left eye closed. Before all of his medical problems started, Paul had loved reading the newspaper and would do so avidly every day. Now that had become too difficult, so he didn't bother. We had been to see the eye specialist and he had told us that the nerves had been damaged while Paul was in cardiac arrest and there was nothing that we could do about it. He registered Paul as partially sighted with the Blind Association. The Association would then contact us and talk about what help we could receive for Paul's loss of sight.

As the year went on, I became more and more frustrated by the legal system in general and our legal aid solicitor in particular. To date, she still had not asked us for a full statement of the facts as we saw them and when I would call to inform her of new issues, she would listen to me, but never comment on anything. For example, I told her about the blood tests that the nurse had sent me, but our solicitor had never asked me for a copy. I just held on to them, assuming she would get around to it at some point. She told me that she had asked for updated files from the hospital, but had not received them yet. When I called the director of nursing to ask her why this was, she stated that she had not received any such request from our solicitor. She told me, as she had before, that she had everything ready to send, but that she needed the request first. I was annoyed with our solicitor, but not quite sure what to do, so I let this go on for some time and by then it was August.

I had been leaving messages on the solicitor's voicemail, but she wasn't returning any of my calls. One day I finally got through to her secretary, who politely informed me that I was not the solicitor's only client. I explained I understood that, but needed her to get in touch with the hospital. When I think back on all this, it seems incredible to me that I put up with such incompetence for so long, but what could I do? She did nothing, even after I told her that the hospital had verbally admitted liability. The first thing a good solicitor would have done would be to have got that in writing from the hospital. But when you are on legal aid, you don't have the choices that you would have it you were paying for your own counsel, so I didn't feel that I had the right to complain.

I watched as Paul became slowly more and more depressed at the lack of help and compensation. Finally I couldn't take it anymore. I called the solicitor and told her exactly what I thought of her. I didn't attack her personally, but she represented the system to us and it wasn't working. She apologised and promised to get things moving right away. We accepted her apologies and hoped that things would finally start to get sorted out. We had been told by the hospital to ask for an interim payment to help us out financially. After all this time of not working and all of Paul's special needs, money was getting very tight. I hoped that if we got a few pounds, Paul could get some things he needed to make his life a little easier and then maybe his depression would lift. I told the solicitor that she needed to request the payment and that we needed it urgently. A couple of weeks went by and still I heard nothing about the payment. When I contacted the administration at the hospital, they said that nothing had been requested. I was fed up by now and contacted the firm that our solicitor worked for. I asked to speak to another solicitor, as ours wasn't returning my calls. I was put through to the head of the department. I told him about all of the problems that I had been having and said that I would like to change my solicitor to another one in the practice. He informed me that ours was the only clinical negligence solicitor that they had in the firm and that, although he handled some cases in that field, he wasn't free to take on any more at the time. He was concerned about my allegations and asked my permission to look into things further. Of course I agreed. A short while later, his secretary got back to me saying that he and our solicitor would like to come see me and Paul at home. We arranged the visit for the following week. When they came over, they discussed what they would do to keep our case with them, although they acknowledged that we had every reason to be fed up with them and that they could understand if we chose to find someone else. Our solicitor said that she was sorry that she had let us down, but that she had been very busy and would love the chance to make things up to us. At the time we agreed to give it one more go.

The following week we received a letter from the solicitor confirming the details of the meeting we had at our house. However, by this time Paul and I had talked it over and decided that we needed to find someone else. We simply did not trust her anymore and didn't feel that she had our best interests at heart. We knew that changing solicitors would delay our compensation claim, but we were prepared to wait. I called her up to inform her of our decision. When I told her that we were going to move to another solicitor, I was quite surprised when she bluntly said to me, "you'll find that it's not so easy to change solicitors when you're on legal aid."

"So you're saying that just because we're on legal aid, we don't have any choices?" I asked her, beginning to get just a bit cross.

"Yes," she replied, "that's correct!"

"We'll see about that," I said to her, ending the call. I was amazed at how little she knew about me. Did she think that we had come this far just to let her push us around? I found her behaviour disgusting, considering that she was supposed to be representing us. It infuriated me that she thought she could do whatever she wanted to us, assuming that we were in a vulnerable position and wouldn't be able to fight back.

Trying to rebuild our lives

Now that I had sacked our solicitor, I wasn't quite sure where to turn to for help. I needed some sort of advice and guidance from someone who had experience and was in a position of some authority. I thought about it for a while and decided to contact our MP. I got through to his office and spoke to his secretary. I told him the story and, though I tried to keep it brief, it still took about twenty minutes. He listened to what I had to say and then asked me if I would like to attend that Friday's surgery. I asked him if he could assure me that there would be a mains socket in the room so that if I needed to give Paul suction, I would be able to do so. Realising that they would have difficulty accommodating us, he then said, "maybe it would be better if the MP came to your house to see you?" This sounded very good to me, as getting Paul around was still a bit difficult, especially now that it was beginning to get cold in the evenings and the MP's surgery was at 7.00 pm. The secretary said that he thought the MP would be able to make it in two weeks' time, on the Friday afternoon, but that someone would call me to confirm. I thanked him and said goodbye. The phone rang the following day and it was our MP on the line. He confirmed the meeting for Friday afternoon 7th September. Then I asked him if he could recommend a good solicitor, as we had decided not to stay with the one we had. He advised me to look up the Law Society's list, but then later rang me up with a list of three names that he had come up with himself. I was immensely grateful.

I wanted to have our new solicitor in place by the time our MP came around, so I contacted one of the firms on the list that he had given me and spoke to a lawyer. She listened to our story patiently and then said that she would love to take the case on. We were thrilled – she sounded competent and was very easy to talk to. I copied all of my documents and sent them to her through the mail. She informed our previous solicitors that she had been asked to take over the case and sent in an application to Legal Aid for the transfer. It was quite a blow then the following week, when we got a letter in the mail turning down our request for a transfer. With our request for a transfer denied, it meant that we would have to stay with our previous solicitor. But after all that had happened between us, how could we do that? I called our previous solicitor and she told me that the legal aid authority has the right to refuse a transfer. From what she said to me, I deduced that she had objected to us moving our case. I couldn't understand that at all. She didn't care about us and had done nothing for us, so why did she care if we remained her clients? I called our new lawyer about it as well and she was quite calm. She told me that it was alright and that we would just appeal the decision. I wasn't really sure what all of that involved, but I left it in her hands, since she obviously knew what she was talking about. It was a great feeling to finally have someone competent on your side, someone whom you could trust.

On the 7th September our MP arrived as promised. I made him a cup of tea and then told him our story, with all the gory details. He was appalled at how Paul had been treated in hospital and actually said to him, "I am so sorry Paul". I told him that lack of attention and care were not the only problems and went on to give him the story of the missing blood test results. He was horrified and agreed with us that we had a right to be concerned. He told me that in addition to lawyers, we might have to involve the police at some point, but that he needed to think about this further. From there I went on to our financial situation and how desperately we needed that interim payment. Obviously the main hold-up was the legal aid situation. He was shocked at the behaviour of our solicitors and he called them up there and then. He introduced himself and then told them what he thought about their handling of our case and advised them to let the case go. He informed them that he would be contacting Legal Aid right after he spoke to them. Next he called up Legal Aid, asked to speak to someone in authority and then briefly outlined our case for them. He asked them to change over our legal aid certificate to our new solicitors and they agreed to do so right away. I was so happy, I couldn't stop thanking him. Perhaps finally we could move forward and get some much needed help. I told him that I couldn't believe how easily he could get things done and how hard I had been trying for so long to accomplish the same things. He then said something that I will never forget: "MPs don't have any power, people just don't realise it." We had a good laugh over that and it was nice to see Paul pulling himself up out of his depression for a change, even if only for a little while. Our MP got up to go at that point, telling us that he would be back in touch soon. Once again I thanked him and he left.

First thing Monday morning, I called our new lawyer to tell her that the transfer had been approved. She got on the case right away and contacted the hospital and the NHS solicitors. She told us that she would apply for the interim payment immediately and then begin looking around the country for specialists who could confirm Paul's injuries. She explained that this might take some time, due to the fact that Paul had so many injuries and each required a different doctor. But we were willing to wait – we were just glad that things were finally moving.

It was approaching Christmas and Paul had begun to have some problems with his breathing even through the tracky tube, but we weren't sure what was causing it. There seemed to be obstructions from time to time and he had to go on his nebulizer a lot more often to get relief. We thought that it was probably a plug of dried phlegm stuck in his tube and decided we would just monitor it to make sure it didn't get any worse. He wanted to get something done about his voice, but we weren't sure yet what our options were. He made me understand several times that if he had to live the rest of his life without speaking, then he didn't want to live. I would tell him off, mainly because I could sense that he was serious and it scared me. We had to go to the hospital pretty often for his stump, which was causing him a lot of pain. They had established that it wasn't phantom pains he was suffering from, but probably some kind of nerve damage, which they hoped would settle down in time. Meanwhile, I tried to ease the pain for him by massaging it several times a day. Ironically, now that he had all these other problems, Paul's initial health concerns seemed to have settled down. His arthritis was not causing him much grief and his diabetes had also settled down.

On the 11th October, we had a major meeting scheduled with the hospital. Fortunately, our MP could attend it with us. If all went well, then the matter of our interim payment could be settled there and then. On the day itself, Paul and I went in early as usual to navigate the wheelchair. When everyone had arrived and sat down, the director of nursing did the introductions and then we began to go through a list of questions that we had previously given to her and the chief executive. Many of their answers were confusing to us, but we were assured that the details of what they were saying would be sent to us in a letter afterwards. What became clear during the meeting was that the blood test results from 27th September were still not in Paul's file and neither was the discharge form. I had received signed copies of both, but I had been told by our MP not to show them until our solicitor had commented on them. It seems that even though Paul and I had told the hospital beforehand exactly what we wanted answers to, they were still trying to find ways to delay us.

Included on our list of fourteen questions was Paul's request that he be given a formal apology by the hospital as he thought that would help soothe his mind. We brought that up at the meeting and were told by the chief executive that it was not possible yet, due to the litigation that was going on, but that he would try to include some sort of apology in his letter to us afterwards. We were astounded by this, since they had already verbally admitted blame. It just seemed common decency, after all they had put Paul through, to give him something as simple as an apology if he thought it would help him.

The lectures that we were involved in at the hospital were going quite well and sometimes we did as many as three workshops in one week. The whole hospital was talking about them, but it was still hard for the nurses to get time off their shifts to attend one. During one lecture, a woman cried so much that she had to leave the room. At another meeting, a nurse got very angry with us and didn't believe that what had happened to Paul could have happened at the hospital.

Shortly before the Christmas holidays, the director of nursing came over to our house with our much-needed and long-awaited interim payment of £10,000. This was a great relief as by then we were deep in debt, with no idea of how we could ever pay all our bills. She also gave Paul a medic alert bracelet that we had been promised months earlier. We made the best that we could of

Trying to rebuild our lives

Christmas, but it was hard to tell if things were going to get any better. We still had our dreams of getting a bungalow, but we weren't any closer to it than we had been a year ago. As the New Year came, it was hard not to reflect and compare the way things were now to the way they used to be. Paul and I had decided that we didn't want him to be a burden on our sons. Not that they weren't willing to help, but they were young and deserved to enjoy themselves. He didn't ever want to be in a position where he was dependent on them and where he might ruin whatever future they might have. So we made it seem as though we could cope with everything and actively discouraged them taking a hand in his care. This was all well and good in principle, but it was so hard for me to care for Paul with no relief and no one who I could really talk to about what I was going through. It would have been so nice to know that someone was going to look after Paul for a few hours, maybe take him to a football game or to do some shopping. I just needed to know that for a few hours I wouldn't have to be constantly listening to see if he was breathing. I knew that most people were frightened to offer to look after him, because they wouldn't know what to do if something went wrong when they were with him. Paul's amputation clinics had stopped by now, as there was nothing more for him to learn. So I didn't even get that break anymore. Paul had got quite close to several of the men in the class, not to mention the ambulance drivers. It was two mornings of the week that he got to go out and of course he looked forward to it too. I spoke to the hospital to see if I could get him back into them, but they told me that they couldn't let him keep going just for social reasons.

We had already been told by the hospital that Paul could not use his leg outside of the house, as they didn't think it was safe. It probably wouldn't have been possible anyway, as he was in a lot of pain from nerve damage. They recommended that we use it around the house and for cosmetic purposes when we went out. All in all, it was a great disappointment to us. Paul had stopped using it altogether, unless we were going somewhere special where he wanted to look his best. Paul had got used to people seeing him without his leg by now and had even begun to wave to children

142

that we knew with his stump, as a joke. It used to make them laugh and they would ask him to do it again. Once they got past being scared of him, he would have a bit of fun with them and encourage them to look at it and touch it if they wanted to. It was so nice to see that he could still enjoy a bit of life, however small.

On the legal front, it had been established between our MP and the chief executive that an independent enquiry was needed. While we were waiting for news on that, our MP decided that he would like to bring in the police, so he wrote a letter setting out the complaint. Letters had been going back and forth since we had started our claim and it was hard to keep track of all of them. I tried my best but still things got lost. I believe that some people still wanted to cause confusion and so things were being "lost" at the hospital's end or "not received." Paul's case was a big embarrassment to them and now that they had admitted liability, they didn't even want to talk about the fact that he had been dehydrated. Their line seemed to be, "we have admitted liability, so why keep going on about it?" Our new lawyer was beginning to arrange for Paul to see independent doctors for our case against the NHS. Even though they had admitted liability, we still needed to get all of Paul's injuries documented. At the beginning of the year, we had been contacted by the Blind Association and they were scheduled to come out and assess Paul in February.

Breathing had become more and more difficult for Paul over the last few weeks. We were told that it was due to granulation in his windpipe, caused by the tube rubbing excess skin away. One of the doctors had let me look down the fibre optic camera when they were examining Paul and it looked as if there was a small mass of floating white flesh. It moved along with the flow of air, so as Paul breathed out, it was pulled up and blocked the tube. The obvious conclusion was to insert a longer tube, one that would go past the lump of flesh and push it to one side. That way it wouldn't be sucked into the tube with each exhalation. There was another possibility, which was that they might be able to reconstruct Paul's windpipe by using bones from his ribs to reconstruct his airway. This is the same operation that they do with premature babies who have had to be on ventilators for long periods of time. However, this was a major operation and, in order to do it, Paul's health would have to improve substantially.

The doctors had already established that Paul had a subglottic stenosis. I overheard them talking about it. At first I had no idea what they meant. I jotted it down on a piece of paper, so I could look it up later. I did that often if they used a term between themselves that I didn't understand. Rather than wasting time and asking them there and then, I would jot it down on whatever piece of paper was handy and sometimes on my hand or Paul's if there was no paper around and then I would look it up on-line when I went home. That way I could come back and discuss it with them later and I would be a bit more informed. There must have been dozens of little scraps of paper in my handbag with medical terms written on them. As my knowledge of medical terminology grew, doctors and nurses who didn't already know me would sometimes assume that I had a medical background and was perhaps a nurse myself. They would ask me and I would just say "no" and leave them wondering how I knew the things that I did. It was quite fun at times.

Paul was called in for yet another appointment. At first the doctor gave Paul's airway a thorough examination, which involved sticking a tube up Paul's nose and down into his throat. The doctor wanted to get an idea of whether or not he would be able to take the tube out eventually, so he suggested to Paul that they do a CT scan of his throat. Paul agreed. Of all the abilities that he had lost, he missed speech the most. If there was any chance at all that he could get the tube out and be able to speak one day, then he would do whatever was necessary.

On 2nd April, I received a phone call from a police detective. He told me that they had received a letter from our MP and that he had been assigned to look into the allegations. He arranged with me to come to our home in two days time along with a colleague. I knew the story by heart, but I still had a lot of work to do getting the papers in order. Accusing a hospital of tampering with a patient's medical file is a serious matter and I wanted to be able to prove whatever it was I was going to say. The 3rd was a

144

Trying to rebuild our lives

busy day as, in addition to getting the paperwork in order, Paul had three doctors' appointments that I had to take him to.

On the morning of the 4th April, the two policemen arrived. They had warned us that their business would take several hours, so I had prepared a simple lunch for all of us. We all sat down and I began to tell the story. There were certain parts where I always cried and today was no exception. The detective wrote everything down as we went along and asked for the blood test results and other paperwork. When I was done, he told me that he would have to go back to the police station and rewrite everything, then bring it back some time the next week for me to sign and that would be my official statement. As I was talking, I could see the two policemen looking over at Paul from time to time. I suppose they weren't yet used to the fact that he couldn't speak and were waiting for him to jump in and say something. I know Paul would have loved to have been able to. Sometimes Paul would contribute by reminding me to add details that I had missed or giving points that I hadn't thought of, but he always had to do everything through me. Perhaps if he could have written things down or maybe kept a journal like I did, that would have made things easier for him. But his dyslexia made that very difficult and he was just too embarrassed about his writing to do more than jot down a few words at a time. Paul asked me to tell the two police officers about his wanting to die, so I mentioned it when we were talking after lunch. The detective got up at that point and walked over to Paul. He took his hand and said, "I hope you're alive to see the end results of this investigation." The detective thought that, in addition to the removal of the blood test results, we probably had a case against the chief executive personally. This was because I had contacted him directly about taking certain precautions for Paul, his office had acknowledged my letter and given me their assurances and then not done anything about it. Paul and I both felt safe in the hands of these two officers and reassured by the fact that they seemed angry and horrified by our story.

The speech therapy department at the hospital had given Paul a light writer computer. It was a keyboard where you could type in the word you wanted to use, press play and it would say it

Trying to rebuild our lives

for you. Paul was very eager to try it out and for a couple of weeks he kept it right by his chair and often used it. But obviously his dyslexia was a problem, as the computer would get confused if the word wasn't spelled exactly right. Plus Paul was a very spontaneous speaker and by the time he had managed to type in everything he wanted to say, everyone around him would be talking about something else. Sadly he realised that it wasn't going to give him back his ability to communicate.

The granulation in his windpipe was making Paul cough and at times it would get very bad. There was one night that I will never forget and I still have nightmares about it. He woke up coughing and tried to sit up, not realising that the force of the coughing had burst the tracky collar and the tube had come out. I woke up to see his horrified face and his hand pointing at his throat. It was what he had feared most – he was suffocating. I ran around to him and tried to push the tube back in, but the granulation was blocking the entrance and it wouldn't go. Blood started to pour out and soon it was all over Paul's front and my hands and splattered on my front as well. I rushed into the bathroom to get some sterile tubing and pushed that down into his windpipe. It was a bit thinner than his usual tracky tube, so it fit and once again Paul could breathe. We both started crying with relief, we had been so terrified. We normally didn't like to involve the boys in caring for Paul, but I had been so scared that Paul was going to die that I had yelled out for them to come. While I cleaned everything up, Adam stayed with Paul to make sure that he didn't stop breathing again. I'm sure that the boys were very shaken at the sight of their parents covered in blood in the middle of the night.

I had to replace the tracheotomy tube, because the sterile tubing wasn't the right size and, if I left it in there too long, Paul would begin to have problems breathing again. He kept begging me not to put it back in, because he was afraid that it wouldn't fit and he would suffocate. He looked so pitiful and I was so angry at the NHS for reducing him to this state and for putting his life in my hands. What would have happened if I hadn't been able to get that sterile tubing into his throat? Then he would have died and I would have had to live the rest of my life knowing that I had inadvertently

Trying to rebuild our lives

caused my husband's death. I couldn't understand how hospitals could send someone home with such severe disabilities as Paul had and expect that their families, who had no prior medical training, would be able to take care of them twenty four hours a day. It wasn't just Paul's health that I was concerned about at this point, it was mine as well. Sometimes I didn't think I would be able to take the pressure and stress anymore. It never let up.

At around this time, I began having nightmares about Paul's amputations as well. I would wake up terrified that the doctors were back to cut something else off and I would look around trying to find some way of stopping them. Of course, once I woke up I couldn't go back to sleep again for a long time because all these thoughts were still running around my head. I would lie there reliving the nightmare of him coming out of theatre without his leg and the voice in my mind screaming "sew it back on!" over and over. My memories were so vivid that it was like being there all over again. I still couldn't believe that all of this had happened to us.

Shortly after the episode of Paul's tube falling out, I spoke to a doctor at the hospital. I told her what had happened and she suggested that we put in a softer tube called a Moors. It would go down further as well, so that it would cover the granulation. She told me to bring Paul in the following day. After the doctor examined Paul, she agreed to change to a Moors tube, but wanted to do it in theatre. That way everything would be sterile and if anything went wrong and Paul needed to be resuscitated, it would be easy to do. We also thought that Paul would be safer this way and the date was set for 20th May. Paul was very scared about anything to do with his tracheotomy. He told me that by this point he was no longer afraid of dying, but he was frightened about how he would die. Suffocating was one of his worst fears. I think that this fear led him in part to want to take his own life, so that at least he would be in control of how he died. He could not longer walk, talk or breathe on his own, but at least he could do this one last thing for himself. We went into hospital on the appointed day and Paul and I kissed goodbye as they wheeled him down to theatre yet again. Nowadays, every time we said goodbye we were aware that

Trying to rebuild our lives

it might be the last. No anaesthesia was needed, as the procedure was very simple, so at least that was one thing we didn't have to worry about – Paul being put to sleep and not waking up. About ninety minutes later, a nurse came over with a great big smile to say "he's on his way up." Everyone in the ward knew our history by now and so understood why I wanted to be kept up to date at all times.

Paul had quite a cough when he was wheeled back in, but I was told this was perfectly normal given that his tube had just been changed. He was propped up to ease the coughing, but it didn't seem to be helping much. As time went on, Paul's cough got worse and he started bringing up blood with it. They realised that the tube was going right to the end of the oesophagus, where it divided into two to go into the lungs, and rubbing against the end of it. This was causing Paul to cough and bring up blood. The surgeon was called and what should have been a fairly routine procedure was rapidly becoming an emergency. The Moors tube was quickly taken out and a temporary tube inserted. They tried to taper the new tube a little so it didn't quite touch the end of the windpipe, but when it was re-inserted, Paul still coughed violently. In the end it was decided that the new tube just didn't suit him and the previous type of tube was put back in. The doctor wanted Paul to stay in overnight because of all the coughing and blood loss. Paul wasn't happy about this, but he knew it was for the best and agreed, as long as they would let him go home first thing in the morning. I went home in the afternoon for a few hours, then went back to keep Paul company until he fell asleep. It was about 11.00 pm when I finally left the hospital that night and I came right home and fell into bed, exhausted and frightened. Whenever I was around Paul, I tried my best to seem confident and experienced, but I certainly wasn't feeling that inside. I just didn't know what was going on and was extremely confused. The last two years were beginning to wear me down and I would often cry myself to sleep at night, praying to God to send someone to help me.

They finally decided that the granulation had to come out and an appointment was made with a surgeon. He brought his anaesthetist with him to our appointment. They took out Paul's

148

Trying to rebuild our lives

tube and looked down his windpipe with a fibre optic camera. We listened as the two doctors discussed the difficulty of keeping Paul ventilated while the granulation was removed and how he would bleed profusely. This meant that the blood would need to be suctioned out of Paul's lungs at the same time. Also they were worried that there wasn't enough room in Paul's windpipe to perform the operation. The surgeon told Paul that he wanted to look at the CT scan they had done the previous time Paul had been in hospital and then he would get back to us with his decision. We thanked them and left, feeling a bit disappointed, but still hopeful that he would decide it was safe to go ahead. We never heard anything from the surgeon again. We eventually asked one of his assistants about it and she simply said that the surgeon had decided that the operation couldn't be done. I suppose he had passed on his decision to them, but Paul and I both thought that the least he could have done was to tell us personally about what decision he had made and his reasons for making it.

Following this, Paul started to believe that the doctors had decided not to do anything more for him and that they would let him to die, gasping for breath. He asked me how they could leave him like that when they were the ones who had put him in that position in the first place. I tried to reassure him, but I believed that he was right. I think so much damage had been done to Paul, that the doctors were afraid to touch him in case something else went wrong. I found it disgusting that they put their reputations before a patient's life, especially when it was the NHS that had so badly damaged that patient.

The police had begun their investigation by interviewing the doctors who were involved in Paul's treatment. I quickly learned how lonely it can be when you have some sort of case against another individual or individuals. It was hard to gather information, as everyone I spoke to was worried that I would try to implicate them as well. They would all listen to my story, because they wanted to know everything that I did, but they were not so keen to give me information. They all seemed to be protecting themselves.

Trying to rebuild our lives

The detective had called me to tell me that they had tracked down the doctor who had been on call the evening that Paul was re-admitted, after having been discharged in renal failure. He was a junior doctor and worked for a female consultant who was married to the doctor who had discharged Paul in renal failure. So Paul had been wrongly discharged by one doctor and readmitted into the care of that doctor's wife. And then Paul's blood test results had 'disappeared'. I began to get terrified by the implications of what I was hearing.

It was getting easier and easier for me to talk to people about Paul wanting to die. I suppose sometimes I used it as a lever to try to get people in the system to move a bit faster and get things sorted for us. I wanted to convince them of how bad things really were. But I don't think I ever believed that Paul would take his own life. One day Paul came to me and requested that we sit the boys down and tell them of his desire to take his own life. He didn't think it was right that everyone else knew about it and they did not. At first I was very much against the idea. I thought they were far too young to be able to cope with something like that and they had already been through so much. I also thought that if the boys knew, then it would be much more likely that Paul would actually carry out his plan. Up until then, I had still clung to the hope that Paul was just a bit depressed and would get over it and learn how to live with his disabilities.

Paul kept talking about it over the next few days, saying that he thought they were old enough and responsible enough to deal with the news. He didn't want to take the chance that they would hear about it from someone else. It was also important for him to see what their reaction would be. I think he was afraid that they would think he was a coward and that he was taking the easy way out. Or even worse, that maybe he didn't love them enough to keep on trying. He wanted to make sure that they knew how much he loved them and that he had made this decision because he just couldn't live with what he had become any longer. Deep down, I knew he was right, but I couldn't think of a good way to broach the topic. After all, it was me who would be doing the talking, not Paul

Trying to rebuild our lives

directly. How do you sit in front of your children and tell them that their father wants to kill himself? I told Paul that this wasn't something that I could plan and that we would know the right moment when it came. It would have to be a very casual setting, like one day when we were all watching TV or something. He agreed as long as I didn't let it wait too long. He wanted to get it off his chest. He hadn't planned yet when or how he would do it, but he wanted to make sure that we were all prepared before he thought about that.

I remember when I had told Vanessa and Steve about Paul's wish. We were in the town centre – I took Paul there every Saturday to go to the market. We would walk around for a couple of hours, getting whatever we needed and then have lunch. It was nice for him to get out of the house for a bit. It was nice for both of us, in fact. Sometimes we would run into people we knew while we were out and this particular day it was my sister and brother-in-law. Vanessa suggested that we get a cup of tea as there was a nice little café around the corner and it was a lovely day, so we could sit outside. While we were sitting around the table laughing and joking, Paul kept tapping me, wanting me to break the news to them. I felt physically sick, my stomach was churning and my throat was dry. I couldn't believe that he wanted me to ruin a perfectly nice day like this and I had no idea how they would take it as they both loved Paul dearly. But he kept after me to do it, so eventually I just blurted it out. "Paul wanted me to tell you that he doesn't want to live anymore." There was stunned silence and it went on for what felt like several minutes. Finally Vanessa asked, "why?"

Paul asked me to tell them that he just wasn't happy anymore, trying to live in the mess that they had made of him.

"But how can you want to die after all that you have been through?" Vanessa asked and she seemed almost angry.

I don't remember Steve saying anything at all through this whole thing, but then I was so nervous the whole time that I might very well have just forgotten. It was ironic, because I had felt the same way that Vanessa did when Paul first told me of his intentions and now I found myself having to back him up. "Try to look at it from Paul's point of view," I said. "Of course I don't want him to do it either, but I am trying to understand how he feels." I still felt sick and at that point, I also felt angry with myself. Why was it becoming easier for me to understand that my husband wanted to kill himself and to tell other people? Did this mean that I thought he should do it? I couldn't picture my life without him, but I also didn't know how much longer I could stand to see that lost, sad expression in his eyes or how much longer I could continue to take care of him with very little help from anyone else.

That was the first time I had to tell family members about Paul's wish to die. Somehow I thought that it was going to be a lot more difficult to tell Adam and Lee. But it had to be done, so one day when they came home from work, I asked them what their plans were for the evening. As it turned out, they were both staying in, so I thought that I might as well get it over with. After dinner I told the boys that Paul and I wanted to talk to them about something. They seemed very nervous and I wasn't sure how I was going to break the news to them. Adam and Lee sat on the sofa, Paul was in his remote control armchair and I was opposite him in my lounge chair. It took a while for me to work up the nerve to speak, but finally I said, "your dad has asked me to tell you both something." Then I just dived in, "since your dad has been damaged like this, he just doesn't want to live anymore." I could see the shocked looks on their faces and I hurriedly continued, "he loves us all very much, but he doesn't like his life the way it is now and he is very worried about what he and the rest of us will have to go through in the future." Adam began to cry and Lee just sat there looking stunned. I suppose we had done a good job of keeping our feelings from them, because it seemed that they had never considered this possibility.

Adam looked at his dad then and asked the same question that Vanessa and I had at first. "How can you want to die after all that you've been through?" Paul started crying at that point and then I couldn't hold the tears back either. He looked over at me and wiping his eyes mouthed, "can you tell them for me?"

152

Trying to rebuild our lives

I began by stating the obvious, which was that Paul wasn't happy living with all the damage that had been done to him. Adam quickly jumped in with "but things will be done to correct some of that damage!" Paul shook his head and I said, "your dad doesn't think that any of the doctors are going to risk helping him because of all that he has already been through and because he is so high-risk. They are afraid of ruining their own careers if anything else goes wrong." At Paul's prompting, I went on to say, "your dad feels that maybe if he could talk, he would want to go on living, but he feels so lonely and isolated and scared as well."

Adam was still crying and you could see he was trying to come up with arguments to change his father's mind. "Well, once you get your compensation money, we could go to America and see if a surgeon there could help us," he suggested. Paul shook his head again. "That was a long way off," he mouthed, "if it happened at all." He told them that he didn't intend to end his life right there and then, but that at the moment that was the way he was feeling and he had wanted them to know that. He felt that he owed them at least that much.

Adam drew his knees up to his face by now, to try to hide his tears. Lee still hadn't said anything at all, bless him, he was still in shock. But the look on his face said more than enough and I had to leave the room. I couldn't stand seeing my husband and both my sons so emotionally wrecked. I felt helpless and most of all angry that we were not getting any help from anywhere else either.

Later that night Paul asked me, "do you think they think I'm a chicken?" I would have laughed at how ridiculous that idea was if it wasn't such a serious question.

"How could anyone ever think you're a chicken after all that you've endured. Don't be silly, you are the bravest man I have ever met and I am sure that they think that too."

"I just hope they understand," he mouthed to me.

I looked at him and tried to explain how I felt, without making him think that I was approving his decision. "It's hard for most people to understand, Paul, because they don't have to live in your body. Most people would think, like I did originally, that as long as you have breath left in you, then life is worth living. But I can see what a struggle you go through every day and how you are scared that every breath might be your last. Even if the boys don't understand right now, they will eventually. Most of all, we will just have to learn to respect that it was your decision." I wanted to add something like, "but we still don't want you to go, so please don't do it." But I had already said all that and I didn't want him to feel guilt on top of everything else that he must be feeling. I wondered how much a person has to suffer before they give up and feel that it isn't worth going on anymore. I had been with him every step of the way and even I couldn't really know what he was going through. It hurt me more than I can say that Paul had reached that point. A black cloud hung over us from that day on. We were never really sure when Paul would decide to end things and it was rare that any sunlight got through the gloom.

It was approaching June and we were hoping to hear from social services soon. We had been waiting months and I remained hopeful that maybe, if we could just get a bit of help, then that would make Paul's life easier and he would want to stay with us. He used to love our home before all of this happened, but now he hated being inside our house. He felt trapped and missed the garden that he could no longer go out to. He hadn't even been able to go upstairs since all of this had happened. And he was afraid to let me go upstairs, because then I might not be able to hear him if he started to suffocate. The upstairs rooms only got cleaned when Adam or Lee were around to stay with their father.

A few days later, Paul asked me if I could get some information about living wills for him and also on how to give me power of attorney so I could continue fighting for him if he wasn't able to give his consent. He had also stated his wish not to be resuscitated if he ever went into a coma again. He was very firm about that. He was beginning to get serious about his intentions and it scared me. He wanted me to talk to our solicitor about all this, but I wasn't quite sure whether or how to go about it. I knew Paul wanted all the paperwork put into place, but I was concerned that if I helped with that, in a way I was giving him the go-ahead to kill himself.

Trying to rebuild our lives

I told him that I wanted to see things through to the end with him and that I intended to be there, holding his hand, when he died. He told me that he wouldn't let me, because if he took his own life and I was there, then it would be seen as assisting him and I would be in trouble with the law. That was the most ironic thing I had ever heard in my life. When all the people, who had done things to harm Paul, were getting away without punishment, I his wife, who loved him more than anyone else, might face legal action just because I didn't want him to die alone. I told Paul that I didn't care and that if I got in trouble with the law for loving my husband, then so be it. He knew that once I had made up my mind there was no going back, so he didn't try to change my mind anymore. On some level I hoped that, if he thought I would get in trouble, this might keep him from doing it. After all, with him gone, the boys would need me.

All this time, I had trouble controlling my emotions. Sometimes I felt sorry for him, while at other times I was angry with him. I understood why he wanted to die, but wasn't his family worth fighting for? Didn't over twenty four years of marriage count for anything? We had had our ups and downs like everyone else, but we had always had a strong marriage and a strong family. Where had that gone? How could he suddenly decide something as important as this and then leave the rest of us to deal with it? Perhaps I was being selfish, but I didn't care anymore. I had always had to pretend to be the strong one, but inside I was terrified.

I didn't get around to speaking to our lawyer immediately. Things were continuing to drag out on the legal front. Paul had been to see two doctors for his case against the hospital. But the solicitor told me that he would probably have to see four more. Each one had to read his extensive medical file before meeting with him, so it didn't look like things were going to get sorted out that year.

The police were also apparently having problems. They said they couldn't track down some of the doctors who were involved. The junior doctors had moved all over the country and the one whose signature they thought they had on Paul's discharge form, the one when he was released in renal failure, was believed to be in Africa. The NHS told us that they couldn't be sure whose signature it was exactly and I wondered just why they made doctors sign forms anyway, if it never amounted to anything. This also surprised me as I had a copy of Paul's discharge form and I could clearly read the signature and I knew precisely which doctor had signed it. Moreover, I knew that this doctor wasn't in Africa at all – the doctor was now working in Birmingham.

Dozens of people had been involved in Paul's medical care and where were they now? If it was a cover-up, I couldn't see how it was any more practical from the NHS's point of view than just admitting blame and giving us something to make our lives a little easier. Surely they would have to pay a fortune in legal fees, not to mention what they would suffer if the story ever went public. Why not just make sure our needs were met so that we wouldn't have reason to complain? Why did they seem to be trying to make things as difficult for us as they could? And why put us through so many problems when our family had already suffered so much?

Chapter 12

The mistakes continue

Paul had always had his flaws, we all do and there were times in our marriage, before any of this happened, when he could be quite difficult. He had a wonderful sense of humour, but sometimes his wit could be biting and none of us enjoyed being on the receiving end of it. He would often say hurtful things to me or one of the boys, to the point where they might not speak to him for days at a time. I suppose these things happen in most families, but most families are not as sorely tested as ours was being then.

Since he almost died, Paul had been very grateful to be alive and grateful to have such a loving family around him. Naturally, we were very glad to have him still with us, even in his present state and we all pulled together as a family. Of all the bad things that had happened to us, this one good thing had come out of it. But now that seemed to be ending as well. Paul began to get aggressive and would pick fights with me or Adam or Lee, whoever happened to be around. He now began to take me for granted, whereas at first he had always been very appreciative of everything I did. In his condition, it was all perfectly understandable, but that didn't make it much easier to deal with, especially for me, who was forced to bear the brunt of it.

In addition to our legal battles and Paul's existing medical problems, he had also recently begun to have stomach pains. He described it as an ache on the right side of his stomach that radiated to his back. He had to go to the toilet at least ten times a day to move his bowels and, as it was so hard for him to get around, I can only imagine that this made his mood a lot worse. One specific reason for his anger was that I hadn't yet spoken to our lawyer about his intention to commit suicide. I began to realise that, much as I didn't want to encourage him in taking his own life, I would have to talk with her as it was becoming increasingly obvious that Paul was serious about his plans. Besides, I could no longer take his harassment on the topic and wanted to have some answers and advice myself. Our lawyer was shocked when I did finally get her on the phone, but quickly collected herself and tried to soothe me. She told me that many people in Paul's position would have such thoughts and that it didn't necessarily mean that it would lead to anything. She told me that she would have to get back to me about my specific legal questions as she wasn't a criminal solicitor.

The lawyer rang me a couple of days later and said that the firm she worked for employed someone who was willing to do Paul's living will for him. She also said that she had been speaking to our barrister and that he had agreed with her that we should get a care company involved so that Paul could be properly looked after at home. I was relieved that finally I would be getting some help and trained medical help at that. She told me that she would be calling a private care company and they would come to assess Paul to see what sort of care he needed. We would then approach the NHS with a request for a further interim payment to cover the cost of this care while our claim was being settled. Now it amazed me how much a solicitor could help you, provided you had a competent one, and I was so happy that we had made the move to get a new one. Who knows where we would be had we stayed with our original legal aid solicitor. Needless to say, Paul was quite pleased to hear all of this.

The following week, our lawyer came to see us, along with a lady from the care company. The lady was obviously a seasoned professional. She was introduced to us and immediately pulled up a chair and sat next to Paul, holding his hand. She addressed all her questions to him and let him know that he did not need to speak through me. She could read his lips and understand all of his responses without any of my help. She had clearly been in this sort of situation countless times before and even without my explanations already knew what most of his medical needs were.

The mistakes continue

She told him that she would recommend a few top doctors to him, from all around the country, who might be able to help with the granulation. When she had finished speaking to Paul, she turned to us and explained that the granulation made Paul very vulnerable and that he would need twenty four hour care because of that. This would involve five people, as well as a case manager. They would need me to be on board for the first few weeks, until Paul learned to trust them and they became familiar with his needs, but after that she didn't want me involved in his medical care. I had a family to run and she knew that I needed to get back to being a wife and a mother. The lawyer informed her that she would need to have preliminary report in order to request the funds, followed soon after by a proper assessment and full report.

After they left, Paul told me that he felt very safe with her and was beginning to feel more confident about his future. Hearing that filled me with the hope that maybe we did have a chance after all. I couldn't wait to have a bit of time to spend with the boys and maybe some for myself as well. Perhaps our lives could get back to normal. Nevertheless, a few days later we were phoned by our lawyer's colleague and we discussed what Paul wanted in his living will. We particularly wanted to know the implications of me being with him when he committed suicide. It was decided that a letter would be written freeing me from any responsibility in his death. We were told that it wouldn't be a legal document, but that there was no harm in having it done, as at least it would express Paul's intent and sentiments.

Paul continued to complain about his tummy trouble and, even though he had been given some medication, it didn't seem to be helping him at all. He asked if I would go and see our family doctor. So I made an appointment for myself, making sure that Adam and Lee would be home when I went, as Paul still could not be left on his own. I had made Paul promise me that he would not kill himself when he was alone with one of the boys, but I still got incredibly nervous every time I left him with them. Morbid thoughts about him going into the bedroom and taking his life would fill my head and it was becoming very stressful for me. I

The mistakes continue

told Paul repeatedly that if he did that, it would scar them for life. I'm not sure whether or not he agreed with me, but he did promise that he wouldn't do it.

At first, I talked to our doctor about Paul's stomach problems and then went on to his suicide wish. I became very emotional and broke down in the middle of the discussion. I knew that asking him to give Paul advice on such a serious issue was not part of his job, but I knew how much Paul respected him and felt comfortable enough with him to do this. At the end of our meeting, he told me that he would come by the next day to talk to Paul. I thanked him and left.

When the doctor arrived the next morning, he began by talking to Paul about his stomach trouble and wrote him out a prescription for peppermint. As Paul was already being treated by a consultant for this problem, there wasn't much else that our GP could do without first talking to the other doctor. This discussion didn't take very long and when it was over, our GP asked for a chair so that he could sit right near Paul and took his hand. "What's this I am hearing about you not wanting to live anymore?" he asked.

"I don't want to live this way anymore," Paul replied. "I'm not happy. And I'm scared."

"Of course you are scared and it is normal to feel that way. But things will get better. They already have, haven't they? I don't know what religion you are, but it's not your choice when you die. God is the only one who can choose that, not you." Paul just nodded at him and smiled, so the doctor continued, "I am being serious Paul, lots of people worked very hard to make you better, so you should want to live on."

"I know that people did their best to make me better," Paul answered, "but they didn't know how I would end up at the time. They had no idea that I wouldn't be able to walk, talk or breathe for myself anymore. My life is not worth living."

"It still doesn't give you the right to end your life," the doctor insisted. Paul simply shrugged his shoulders. "I don't want to hear you talking of this again," the doctor said and concluded

The mistakes continue

the conversation. He got up to go and I walked him to the front door. "He'll be OK," he said to me, "he's just a little bit depressed. That is normal given the circumstances. Speak to his consultant at the hospital and see if he has any more advice to give you." With that, he left.

When I went back in, Paul just looked at me and mouthed, "no one understands. I need to be given hope about my future, not talks about what God wants." There was a brief pause before he continued, "mind you, even people that did give me hope never actually came back with any. They promised things and then either never got back to me or managed to back out in some way."

I couldn't think of anything to say. To be honest, I was beginning to lose hope in people too. Paul's face looked so sad these days and somehow it made his injuries look more severe. I often thought the mental abuse that the hospital and NHS were inflicting on us was even worse than the physical abuse that Paul had suffered. At least they were doing something to treat the physical symptoms, but they were doing nothing at all to relieve our emotional suffering. Paul began to speak again. "Do you think they are just taking their time hoping that I will die before they have to pay out? All the solicitors and doctors involved in my case are earning lots of money out of it and being paid straight away, whereas the one person who needs it, me, is still suffering."

I didn't want to answer Paul right away because I needed time to think and anyway I didn't want to risk making him even angrier or more depressed. That was the last thing that he needed. But what he had said was the only thing that really made sense. Why else would they be taking so long to reach a decision in our case? Probably they were just hoping that if they ignored us, we would go away.

Paul's stomach pain continued to worsen over the next few days and his belly began to swell. He refused his food, which caused problems because of his diabetes. His blood sugar level began to go haywire and I had to try my best to convince him to have little bits of things to eat. One day the pain got so bad, that he began to cry and kept asking, "why me?"

The mistakes continue

I tried to comfort him, but I didn't know what was wrong and there wasn't really much I could do. He had undergone several tests for his bowels by this point, but they didn't show that there was anything wrong. I encouraged him to eat, not only because of his diabetes, but also because the painkillers wouldn't be very effective without food. He continued to get worse though and later that day began to have very bad diarrhoea, which was green in colour. He asked me to promise him that I wouldn't take him to the hospital, but I told him that I couldn't do that. I couldn't treat him if I didn't know what was wrong and if he got worse, then I would have to take him back to the hospital. I felt so sorry for him that he had to face the idea of being readmitted to the place that had already caused him so much damage, but there was nothing else that I could do. I remember it was over the weekend that he got much worse. He refused to take his pills on Saturday or Sunday and didn't even drink his proper amount of water. I knew I couldn't let him go on like this much longer. I told him that if he wasn't better by Monday morning, I would have to do something about it.

I wasn't sure what to do though, so I waited until after 9.00 am on that Monday 14th June and then called the director of nursing. Although she had let us down several times, with disastrous results, I needed some advice and could not think of anyone else I could ask. I began telling her about Paul's symptoms, but I got so upset halfway through my description that I started crying. I was really having a hard time coping with this new illness and desperately needed someone to help me. My crying obviously made her aware of this and she said to me, "Mandy, listen to me. I'm sending an ambulance for Paul now, so just get him ready. I will see the two of you when you get into casualty." I just said OK and thanked her, relieved that someone else was taking control.

By this time, Paul wasn't in a fit state to resist as the pain had become so bad. The ambulance arrived within fifteen minutes and I could relax slightly as trained medical staff took over from me. I had got used to taking care of Paul's tracky and stumps and managing his arthritis and diabetes, but still I wasn't a doctor or

The mistakes continue

nurse and I wasn't comfortable treating him for illnesses that I knew nothing about and had received no training for. We received immediate attention when we arrived in casualty, with several doctors coming right over to look at Paul. After a brief examination, Paul was admitted to a ward to have some tests done and given morphine to alleviate the pain.

The doctors thought that gallstones were the likely cause of Paul's pain, but the green diarrhoea meant that there was also some sort of infection. Because of the infection, Paul would have to be on a barrier, which meant that none of us were allowed to touch him without first putting on gloves and an apron. We would have to wash our hands before going into his room and also upon leaving it. With someone in his condition, simple infections could be deadly.

The director of nursing came in to see us at around 11.00 am and was brought up to date on Paul's condition. She told us that she would find a ward that was capable of handling Paul's needs and then returned shortly after to tell us that she had got him a private room on a ward that specialised in elderly patients and stroke victims. I had heard that the staff there were very caring, so I didn't see any reason why it wouldn't be appropriate for us. A porter came to wheel Paul over to the ward and as we were going to our room, we passed some very sick older people. Paul's room was right behind the nurses' station, which was reassuring as they would be able to monitor him much more closely. But when we went into the room, we saw that it had not yet been prepared – there was blood splattered on one of the walls and faeces on the curtains that surrounded the wash basin. I was a bit disgusted, but didn't say anything, assuming that they just hadn't had time to clean it up yet.

They wheeled Paul's bed over to the window, put the brakes on and then began tidying up a bit and putting his personal items in the cupboard. I began to get nervous, as it was obvious that these members of staff had no idea what Paul's medical needs were. When they were done, one of the nurses looked at me and

The mistakes continue

said, "OK, he is settled now, so you can go home. Visiting hours start at 3.00 pm."

I was quite shocked. All I could manage to say in return was, "excuse me?"

"Visiting begins at 3.00 pm," she repeated. I don't think she was being hostile, she just had not been told that Paul had special needs and that his health was extremely fragile. I didn't want to cause any problems with her, as I already knew how resentful hospital staff could get if it looked like you were questioning their authority or judgement, so I decided I would just sort things out with the people in charge of the ward.

"Could I possibly speak to a sister please?" I asked her, smiling and trying to make my voice sound as polite as possible.

"The sister isn't here," she responded, "but I can get you a staff nurse."

I told her that would be fine and then sat down to wait. Paul looked over at me and mouthed, "please don't leave me. They obviously don't know about me here."

I smiled at him and said, "don't worry, I'm not going to, ever." I didn't want to upset him, but I was quite angry by then. How could they put him in this ward, when it clearly wasn't equipped to handle someone as ill as Paul? I wasn't even supposed to touch him without putting gloves on and yet there was excrement on the curtains and blood on the walls of his room! The more I thought about it, the more furious I became. The staff nurse arrived about thirty minutes later. Thankfully she had a big smile on her face, because I'm not sure what I would have said to her otherwise. She greeted me and then said straight away, "wow, I can't believe we have you on our ward."

"Yes," I answered, but must have looked puzzled, because she began to explain.

"I came to one of your lectures a while ago and you really changed the way I nurse. I am so proud to meet the two of you. I use your story all the time when I am training our junior nurses, to explain about how to care for patients. Your story really affected my life."

The mistakes continue

"Thank you," I said, smiling at her and feeling a bit flustered at all the attention.

"No, thank you both. I must make sure that everyone knows we have celebrities on our ward!" Even Paul laughed at that and I was glad to see it, because it meant that his pain was starting to ease up a bit.

She explained to us that Paul's tummy trouble was billary pain, which she said was something like colic. She told us that he had been placed under the care of a cardiologist. When she was finished, I began to tell her why I had asked to see her in the first place, which was that Paul felt very unsafe and vulnerable in the room they had put him in. She seemed completely surprised. I began my explanation with, "you see, if Paul were here without me and his tracky tube blocked, he wouldn't be able to do anything."

"Wouldn't he just take the inner tube out?" she asked

"Well, he's got arthritis, you scc, so he doesn't have the strength in his fingers to twist the tube."

"Oh," she said and thought for a moment. "We'll just have to make sure that he always has the call button on his bed," she said smiling.

I knew that she was trying her best, but I couldn't really believe that she thought that would work. "What good would that do?" I asked her. I didn't want to seem rude, but I wanted her to really think about what his condition was and the sort of care that he would need.

"That way he can call us whenever he needs to," she replied

"But that won't work," I said, "you know that it can often take many minutes after the call button is pushed before a nurse has the chance to check on a patient. By that time Paul would have suffocated. He can't even get off of his bed to get your attention because of his leg. There's no way that just having the call button would be good enough."

"You're right," she said, smiling apologetically. "I'm so sorry, I didn't even think of that." She looked around and then came up with another idea. "What we can do is to move his bed around so that he is right next to the red crash alarm button. If he presses that then everyone will come running."

That seemed like a feasible solution to me, so I thanked her and we began to rearrange the room. While we were doing so, I also asked to be able to look after Paul's non-urgent medical needs as his tracky needed to be cleared up to ten times a day and I knew that nurses would not have the time to see to him so often. She understood that I wanted him to be properly looked after, but didn't want to cause the hospital staff too much inconvenience, so she agreed that I should have twenty-four hour access to Paul. It's ridiculous that I should have felt as if I was being a bother to the nurses by wanting proper care for my husband. I told her that our normal routine in the past had been for me to stay with Paul until he fell asleep, between 10.00 and 12.00 at night, and then to return at around 8.00 am when he awoke. She said that was fine with her.

I began to realise that I would never be able to leave Paul alone, unless it was with someone who was specifically trained to care for him. I didn't resent having to take care of Paul, but I did resent the fact that the NHS expected me to do it for free and they were the ones who had caused the damage. Also I was still worried about the excrement on the curtains and the blood on the walls, but I thought that I had asked for quite a lot already. After the staff nurse had left, I approached another one of the nurses about it. Apparently it was an outside company that dealt with the cleaning and the curtains and she told me that she would have to contact them to get them in to sort things out. It seemed strange to me that hospital staff couldn't deal with this kind of problem, but she did seem eager to help, so I just thanked her and left it at that. I began to wash the blood off the wall and as I was doing so, I noticed the suction tube in the wall next to the oxygen tank. It was quite old and had obviously been used – there was dried blood and mucus on it. There was no way I could use that on Paul for fear of infection. So though I was starting to feel like a bit of a nag, I asked one of the auxiliaries if she could get a new one for me. She seemed to think that I was asking a bit much, but she did it anyway. Finally, we were beginning to feel a bit settled and slightly safer.

The mistakes continue

A little before 5.00 pm, a senior house doctor came over to have a look at Paul. He remembered us from Paul's previous stays and was very kind to us, explaining in great detail what they would be doing over the next few days. As they weren't sure what was wrong with Paul, they would have to work it out by a process of elimination using a series of tests. They would keep Paul on morphine for the pain though and as he was already hooked up to a drip, the morphine would be administered by IV. The doctor told Paul that the morphine dose should last about four hours, but that if Paul felt the pain coming back before that time, then he should ask to have another dose. Apparently it's harder to settle the pain once it becomes bad than it is to suppress it. However, morphine itself suppressed breathing, so if Paul was having trouble with that, he should let the nurses know right away. An antidote would be kept in the nurses' locked room and they would be able to give it to him as required. Normally Paul would probably have been quite worried about his breathing, but he had been in such bad pain for the past five days that he was just relieved to have it reduced.

Paul began to settle in, but kept telling me over and over again not to leave him. I promised that I wouldn't. Nurses kept coming in and out that afternoon and evening to welcome us. They said that they had heard all about us and many of them had been to our lectures. Of course we didn't remember all of them from the classes, but it was wonderful to see that we had made an impact on them. It made the first day of being back in hospital a bit more bearable for Paul.

Paul had a morphine shot due at 9.00 pm that first night, but began to feel the pain at about 8:30 pm. He thought he could hold out a bit longer, but by 8:45 the pain had got to the point where he thought he should request the morphine. I went out and spoke to the nurse on duty. She said that she would put a call in to the doctor right away. I went back in to sit with Paul and we were still waiting there ten minutes later, with no doctor in sight. The pain was getting rapidly worse, so I went back out to speak with the nurse. She said that she had put in the call, but that there was only one emergency doctor on duty and she was stuck in casualty.

167

The mistakes continue

She told me that the doctor had promised to get there as soon as possible. When I got back to Paul's room, he was lying on his side facing the wall, just holding his stomach. He wasn't very interested in what I had to say because the pain had become so bad that he couldn't really focus on me anyway. A little while later the nurse came in to see how he was doing. I was furious by then and felt ashamed that I couldn't do anything to help my husband.

"This is ridiculous," I fumed, "he was due an injection thirty minutes ago. The doctor told us this afternoon not to let the pain get a grip or else it would take even longer to settle again. Since there's not doctor here, couldn't you give Paul an injection?"

"I'm sorry," she said, "but when a drug is given intravenously, then it has to be done by a doctor. Nurses can inject the drug subglottic, but then it doesn't act as quickly." She looked at me and must have not been sure if I knew what she meant, because she explained, "sub-glottic means in the backside. But anyway, if it was prescribed as an IV, then I can't change the orders. His doctors would have to do that." I knew that morphine is a very dangerous drug, but I didn't understand why it was prescribed as an IV when they must have known that it's hard to get a doctor over during the night shift. By the time the doctor did get around to giving Paul his injection, it was after 11.00 pm. Both the nurse and the doctor were very apologetic.

I left the hospital at around midnight, feeling terribly ashamed at the way my husband had been treated. Paul had begged me not to bring him back to the hospital and I had. But what choice did I have? Once again I cried myself to sleep that night. The next morning I got to the hospital bright and early at 7:30, hoping that Paul had a good night's sleep and would be well rested and cheerful. I had no such luck though. He had needed another morphine shot in the middle of the night and went through the same problems all over again. He hadn't wanted to wake the whole ward by pushing the crash button, so he had waited until he saw a nurse nearby, then attracted her attention by banging on the cupboard. This time the doctor didn't take quite as long to come,

The mistakes continue

but it was still long enough for Paul to get very distressed by the pain.

He was cross with me for leaving him alone, but I tried to explain once again, that it was impossible for me to sleep on the hospital chairs. I had to go home and shower and see to Sheba and try to get what little sleep I could. I felt so guilty that I couldn't be there for him every minute of the day, but I was doing all that I could and sometimes already felt that I would snap from all the pressure.

A senior doctor came by to see Paul at around 11.00 am and when we told him all that had happened during the night, he was quite embarrassed. He had already been through a lot with us the previous year. He said that he felt awful, because Paul had suffered so much and he had wanted him to be as comfortable as possible. I said that with all the different medicines and pain-killers we have these days, I didn't see any reason why anybody in hospital should suffer like Paul had. We asked the doctor if the morphine could be administered sub-glottic. I had explained to Paul what that meant and he agreed to have it done that way. Even if it took a bit longer to take effect, at least he would be able to get it whenever he needed it and wouldn't have to suffer like he had during the night. The doctor immediately consented and it was written into Paul's chart that he would have morphine via an IV during the day and injected at night. This made us both a lot less nervous. Another good thing that happened towards the end of the day was that the curtain company came to change the curtains around the wash basin. It was such a relief, as we had to sit there looking at them all day and I was always afraid I would touch something infectious when I drew the curtains for Paul to go to the toilet.

They still weren't any closer to finding out what exactly was wrong with Paul though. His stools were still green, so he was still on barrier and he had stopped eating. Because of this, they had put him on a sliding scale for insulin. That meant that it would drip slowly into his blood all day and the nurses would check his blood-sugar level every four hours and then adjust the flow accordingly.

The mistakes continue

They did this by pricking his fingers to get a bit of blood and it got to the point where Paul was complaining that the ends of his fingers were sore. But it was the best way to deal with his diabetes, especially as he couldn't hold down food. After about a week of this, Paul was still in pain, but trying to control it without the morphine. We tried to tempt him with little morsels of food, but even when we could get him to eat something, he would usually vomit soon after. He would even vomit after drinking water sometimes. This was quite scary, as he had been taken off the drip by now and was controlling his own fluid balance.

They still suspected that Paul's pain was caused by gallstones, so the doctor had arranged for a surgeon to come and see Paul. For the next few days, Paul wouldn't let me leave his side, even to get food, in case the surgeon came to see him while I was gone. That meant, in addition to everything else, I had to remember to pack some sandwiches and fruit for myself before leaving for the hospital in the morning. Paul would still have toast waiting for me for breakfast when I got there, just like he always used to. It was hard going, but somehow I coped and it was worth it to see him smile at me when I got there every morning, even though he might be annoyed with me for leaving him alone.

Paul's room was on the ground floor, overlooking the road that led to the maternity car park. That was where I would put the car when I came every morning to see him, so he liked to look out the window and see me passing by on my way in. I suppose it made it seem to him as if I was there a few minutes earlier. The ward was not perfect, but Paul and I developed a very good relationship with the nurses who worked there. Unlike some nurses on other wards, they didn't seem to mind that I was there from early in the morning to late at night. Not only did they understand that I was just concerned for Paul, but they also seemed to welcome my help. We came to trust them and eventually it got to the point where I felt safe if I had to rush off for a few minutes to do something, knowing that I could count on them to look after Paul.

The mistakes continue

Now that Paul had become very ill again, he was determined to get his legal affairs sorted out. He had me contact our lawyer to tell her that he was very poorly and ask if it was possible to get his living will and power of attorney wrapped up as soon as possible. She spoke to her colleague and then got back to me to tell me that he would take the train to the hospital the following Thursday with the documents and that I needed to have three witnesses lined up to sign them. Once the documents were all signed, Paul felt an immense sense of relief that everything was taken care of and I had to admit that it was a weight off my mind as well.

The following day, Adam and Lee came to visit earlier than usual, at around lunchtime. They asked me if I wanted to go and have lunch with them in the restaurant at the hospital, but I told them that I couldn't, as the surgeon was finally scheduled to come and examine Paul that day and I didn't want to miss him. One of the nurses volunteered to keep an eye out for him and to come and fetch me when he got there, but Paul wasn't comfortable with that, as he knew that all of the nurses were busy and it wasn't possible for them to look after him all of the time. Lee then offered to stay with Paul, while Adam and I went to get some lunch, then he could come and fetch me if the surgeon arrived. I was a bit apprehensive, as the restaurant was quite a walk from the ward, but eventually I agreed. It was lovely to get a break and get out of the room a bit and I was looking forward to having a chat with Adam. It wasn't often that I got a chance to chat with either of the boys in those days. We had just sat down to a roast beef lunch, when Lee arrived to say that the surgeon was with Paul. I left Lee to eat with Adam and I ran all the way back to the ward.

I went straight into Paul's room and he didn't look happy at all. I asked him what was wrong, but he wouldn't tell me, he just mouthed that I should go and have a word with the doctor, who was at the nurses' station reading Paul's file. I went out and stood in front of him, trying to get his attention. He obviously saw that someone was standing in front of him, but he refused to look up. Finally I was forced to lean over the counter and say, "excuse me doctor, but could I have a word with you about my husband, Paul Steane?"

He looked up now, but there was no smile on his face. In fact, there was no facial expression at all. My guard immediately went up. "What would you like to know?" he asked, as though it wasn't painfully obvious that I wanted to know what was wrong with my husband.

"Well, first of all, I would like to know what you think the problem with Paul is."

"Most likely it's gallstones, though we won't know for certain until after the ultra sound is done. If it is, then we still have a problem, because Paul is not a very good candidate for surgery."

"What do you mean?" I asked, though I already had a good idea of what was coming.

"I've been looking through Paul's file and obviously with all of the problems he has previously experienced, it is quite possible that he might not survive another surgery. Not many surgeons would choose to operate on a man whose health was so frail. I haven't yet decided whether or not I'd be willing to risk it, but if I decide not to, then I will find you a surgeon who will."

I couldn't believe that he was so brazenly telling me that he might not treat my husband because he was afraid of the consequences to his career if Paul died. He spoke so casually about it, as though there wasn't a human being in great pain lying in the bed and as though that person's life didn't matter when compared to his career.

"But surely you can't leave Paul like this? Surely the patient comes first?" I argued, probably in vain.

"Every surgeon has choices too," he rapidly replied, "if anything goes wrong with a patient, then we have to live with that for the rest of our lives."

"Excuse me," I started to lose my calm, "but it was medical negligence that made Paul a high risk patient in the first place and now you're going to tell me that you're not going to treat him because you would have to live with the guilt if something went wrong?"

The mistakes continue

There were many times during Paul's various stays in hospital and during our dispute with them, when I thought I had heard it all. There were so many things that got me angry or depressed or hurt. Every time something new came up, I would think, 'surely that's the last straw. They couldn't possibly think of something else to say or do to us that would make things worse.' And yet, time and time again, they did manage to find some way to make things worse.

I was quite flustered by this point and I had to force myself to gather my thoughts to listen to what the surgeon was saying. "I see that you have a legal case pending with another hospital," he said, referring to the big white sticker on the front of Paul's file that said "Legal case pending." I just looked at him for a few moments, not really certain what he was referring to. He went on speaking, "this is another reason not to operate. No surgeon will want to go into surgery with a patient who has an on-going case for medical negligence."

I finally realised what he meant. I leaned forward, trying to keep myself from shouting and said to him, "the litigation is not with another hospital, it is with this one! We are here and we still trust people here at this hospital. It seems to me that this has nothing to do with treating Paul, or whether he has gallstones or some other illness. The decision on whether a patient has surgery seems to be based on whether or not it will further a doctor's career and if the patient has on-going litigation, then no one will help him. I have to say that I am disgusted by all of this and I sincerely hope that you didn't say anything like this in front of my husband. He has enough to deal with without knowing that the people who are responsible for his condition now think it is too risky to help him live with it."

He saw that I was upset, so he began to take on a more conciliatory tone. "Of course I didn't say anything in front of your husband, I only found out about the litigation when I came out of his room and started reading his file. Listen, I haven't said yet that I wouldn't operate and if I do decide not to, then I will find you a good surgeon who will do it. What I would rather do now is to leave it for another twenty four hours and see if the pain settles. Then we have to think about when to operate, as it's not a good idea to perform the surgery when the gall bladder is still inflamed. I have to go to Bosnia in September, so if I do decide to do the surgery, it might be best to wait until I've returned and hopefully by then the pain will have settled a bit."

He was obviously just giving me excuses now, so I left him and went to Paul's room to think things through. Like most people, we had to believe what doctors told us because we didn't know any better ourselves. I still trusted what they said, even though they had been wrong so many times. What else could I do? I had no idea about gall bladders and gallstones and whether or not you could deal with them while they were still bothering the patient!

Over the past few years, several of our friends and family members had asked us why we kept coming back to this hospital after all that had gone wrong here. Even Paul sometimes asked me not to bring him back here. But the fact was that we had no reason to believe that this hospital was any worse than any other. Anyway, you have to go where the ambulance takes you. What good would it have done to go to another hospital, even if we had the choice? Besides, by now, most people at the hospital were familiar with Paul and his needs, so at the end of the day, despite all that we had suffered here, Paul and I both felt that he was safest in a hospital where they know him.

I understood that Paul was already anxious after his meeting with the surgeon, so I tried to make light of the situation and not show my own anger. I joked about the roast beef that I had been tempted with, but forced to leave behind. But I could see that Paul wasn't listening to me and that I would have to deal with the issue at hand. So I asked him what was wrong.

"The surgeon has let me know that there is no hope. He said that it might be gallstones, but that even it was, it didn't really matter, because he doesn't think that I would survive the surgery."

I tried to console him. "Paul, he didn't know what he was on about. He didn't realise that the only reason you ended up on life support was because you had been dehydrated. It wasn't your

The mistakes continue

own poor health, it was bad clinical care." But I could see that I wasn't getting anywhere.

"No, I'm not going to make it this time. They are going to let me die."

I hugged him and told him that it wasn't true and when he calmed down a bit, we had a proper discussion about the situation. I told him of my conversation with the surgeon and how angry it had all made me. Paul told me that he really felt as if he had no choices anymore about his life. If he was sick, then he would just be ill-treated and left to die because of all the medical and legal risk surrounding him. No one would help him. He felt he had no option but to end his life, on his own terms. I didn't know how to reassure him, so I told him that I would speak to someone in the chief executive's office the next day and tell them that I didn't think it should be advertised right on the front of Paul's file that his case was in litigation. When I went home that night, I couldn't get the vision of Paul's face out of my mind. He had looked so sad and so scared. I was confused by that, because he looked so scared of dying, yet he kept telling me that he didn't want to live. Perhaps that was why on some level I never really believed he was suicidal.

I called director of nursing the next morning and told her that I needed to meet with her and the chief executive urgently. She agreed to come over to the ward later that day and said that she would phone the sister in charge shortly to let her know what time she would be there. I thanked her and Paul and I waited to be informed about the meeting. Later that day one of the nurses came into Paul's room to tidy up a bit. "Looks like we're having a special visitor on the ward this afternoon," she mentioned in passing.

"Really? Who?" I asked.

"The chief executive of the hospital will be here. We have to clean out all our offices and tidy up the entire ward," she said, only half-jokingly.

I laughed along with her and said, "oh, he's not coming to inspect the ward."

"How do you know that?" she asked.

The mistakes continue

"Because I asked him to come and see me and Paul. We wanted to speak to him about something."

She seemed quite shocked and just said, "oh, really?" She turned to leave us, presumably to tell the rest of the staff not to worry too much. At the door, she looked back and said, "if you see him before we do, could you let us know that he is here?" My face must have shown my confusion because she went on to say, "well, none of us knows what he looks like, we've never seen him before."

When the nurse had left, I got Paul into his wheelchair and we sat near the doorway to his room, just watching everyone bustling about. We noticed that most of the nurses were being a bit quiet with us and we imagined that maybe they thought we had called in the chief executive of the hospital to complain about them. Their minds would soon be put to rest.

When the chief executive and director of nursing arrived, they came into our room and shut the door behind them. They sat down and I brought them both up to date on Paul's condition. I then got down to why I had asked them to come see us. "The reason I've asked you two to come over here is quite a serious one," I began and they both looked at me questioningly. "How is it that someone can be this badly injured by the NHS, but then when he needs help with the medical problems that they have caused, he is denied it because there are big 'litigation' stickers all over the front of his folder? Because of these stickers, doctors don't want to treat him and apparently they have the right to refuse patients care when they don't feel like taking the risk. I thought patients were treated because they were ill. I didn't realise that surgeons were allowed to refuse patients because they were inconvenient to them. Isn't everyone supposed to be equal under the NHS when in need of treatment?"

They looked at one another and all the chief executive could say to me was, "we are both very sorry." He walked to the door, opened it and asked the sister on duty to bring him Paul's medical file. Once he had it in his hands, he simply tore off the label that read 'litigation pending'. "I'll speak to the complaints

The mistakes continue

department and have them come down to speak with you," he said to us, "and will also speak to the doctor concerned."

"Don't bother," I replied, "Paul has already made up his mind about the surgeon. He doesn't want him anywhere near him, ever. Even if it weren't for the litigation, that surgeon made him feel as if there is no hope for him at all. We would appreciate it if you would find another surgeon, perhaps one that will take the time to read Paul's file before seeing him, so that he knows exactly why Paul is in the condition that he's in. We need someone a little more sensitive to Paul's situation."

They apologised again and left shortly after, promising to be in touch soon. The very next day a lady from the complaints department came over to see us. She showed us Paul's file and the changes that she had made to it. There was just a sticker in there now saying that the file was needed by a certain department and that department's name was coded so that nobody but those concerned would know the patient's status. This system would now be put in place for all clinical negligence patients in the future.

The criminal negligence investigations were proceeding at the same time and since Paul was in the hospital for an indefinite amount of time, it was decided that we should just try as best as we could to carry on with what needed to be done. The detective had arranged for one of the doctors involved to come back to the hospital for an interview over the allegations that had been made and this was going to happen the same day. It was arranged to have the interview on the ward because Paul's medical files could not be removed from the ward at the time. The detective promised to come along and see us after the interview. He arrived on the ward and was shown into the meeting. Knowing that he was going to come and speak to Paul and me afterwards, several of the nurses came into our room that afternoon, giggling and asking to be introduced to him. They all thought he was gorgeous. I had to be the bearer of bad news and tell them that he was just recently married.

The interview was finally over at about 4.00 pm and the detective came into our room with all his files to bring us up to

The mistakes continue

date. He started off by saying how sorry he was that Paul was back in hospital and then went on to tell us what an effect our names had on people in the hospital. Apparently there were many staff members who knew our story and wanted to do whatever they could to help us, but there were also others who were afraid of us. I wasn't quite sure how I felt about that, because it was never my intention to frighten anyone or to make people feel unnecessarily guilty. I just wanted the people who had harmed Paul to admit their mistakes and then correct them in the future. Fear makes people turn away and hide, like one nurse who always used to walk the other way when she saw us coming. I didn't want that at all. I wanted people to respect us and treat us with the dignity that all human beings deserved, not do what we said because they were afraid that otherwise we would cause trouble.

Paul had been in the hospital for almost four weeks now and they still weren't sure what was causing all his stomach pain. After one scan, they had even warned us that it might be cancer, as the liver and bowels both showed signs of it. They were hesitant to examine Paul further though, as the tests for cancer were quite invasive and they didn't want to cause more problems than they solved and have Paul end up back on the ITU. For the moment, they were more comfortable just waiting and seeing what happened. Paul was getting very bored and restless being in bed all the time, but at least the pain had settled and he was even off the medication now. He had also been taken off the barrier and was beginning to eat a bit. He asked the hospital if it would be possible for his electric wheelchair to be brought in from home, so at least he would have some mobility. They agreed and he was so excited that he asked Adam and Lee if they would do it that very same day.

The chair was extremely big and heavy and the boys had to get a van to bring it in, but there was no way they would disappoint their dad, so they managed it. They knew how much it meant to Paul, to his dignity more than his feelings of boredom. Up until then Paul had to use a commode, which he hated. Now he would be able to go to the bathroom, not to mention to the shop if he

The mistakes continue

wanted something to eat or drink and even to the coffee shop just for a change of scenery.

After all that he had been through, Paul was not one to sit by and see someone else being abused. We were on a ward for the elderly and, awful as it may sound, they are often the ones who are made to suffer the most, because they are the most vulnerable. Some hospital staff seem to see them more as annoyances than as patients. We saw some quite awful things while we were there and while I don't want to alienate the many doctors and nurses who do truly care about their patients, there are so many out there that don't, that it really quite sickened us to see it. There was the case of an elderly lady, a lovely woman, who was brought onto the ward with little hope of recovery. To everyone's surprise, she did slowly begin to get better though and every time I passed her room, she would smile brightly at me. One morning she kept trying to get the nurse's attention, but it was 8.00 am and they were serving out breakfast so nobody came to see what she wanted. Finally, she managed to attract one of the nurses and ask if they could hoist her onto the commode, as she had to poo. Immediately the nurse replied with, "I hope you're not serious, because we need the hoist to get you out and we are busy doing breakfasts." The patient was obviously embarrassed and explained, "well, I have been waiting a long time and I can't hold it much longer." The nurse, looking very annoyed, went off to find the hoist. She returned a few minutes later without it and informed the lady that it was being used and she would have to wait a little while longer. "OK, I'll try." I suppose being in hospitals for so long had made me a bit suspicious, because I walked over to the bathroom. There was the hoist, with no one using it and no one in the bathroom.

One of the worst examples that I can remember involved an elderly gentleman named Charlie, who was from a farm nearby. He loved to talk and Paul and I would often sit with him while he told us about his family. He had a wife who was in a nursing home and he missed her terribly, but just couldn't take care of her at home anymore. His family brought her to visit him twice and would go off for a coffee so that they could have some time alone to chat.

179

The mistakes continue

They would sit there holding hands and it was the sweetest sight. One morning I arrived a bit after 8.00 am and as I walked past Charlie's bed, I heard him calling for a nurse. I said hello to him and then went in to check on Paul. Paul was very upset and, when I asked him what the matter was, he said, "Charlie accidentally dirtied himself in the night and he has been trying to get a nurse in to clean him up since he woke up, over half an hour ago." They were serving breakfast then and I could see already that they didn't have as many nurses on duty as they normally did. I found out later that two of them had called in sick. As I was helping Paul to wash up, I heard Charlie calling for the nurse several times. The one in charge that particular morning was not the most caring woman and she just kept telling him that he would have to wait. Finally Charlie got so upset that he reached down into his bed and pulled out his hand covered in poo. He held it up so the nurse could see why he was calling her. When she saw it she marched over to him and said, "Charlie, I know you need to be changed, but we can't do that while we are serving breakfast."

Charlie was so upset by then that he started to cry and said, "I can't eat my breakfast either while I'm lying in poo!" He got so distressed that he put his hand to his head. I don't know if he had forgotten that it had poo all over it or not, but either way, it got into his hair. The nurse got very cross with him and grabbed his hand and pushed it back under the sheet. "Keep your hand in there now and I'll feed you your breakfast, then come back to change you." I watched while she fed him. He looked so horribly sad eating his breakfast while sitting in his own filth and with excrement in his hair. But he ate and the nurse took his tray away. Two more hours passed and still no one had come to change him. By now he was begging them for help, constantly waving his hand in the air to get their attention. But the nurse just kept passing him by and saying, "I'll get to you soon." Then 11.00 am came and then it was noon and still he was sitting there in his own excrement. The nurse kept telling him that she would get to him, but meanwhile she had started at the other end of the ward, making beds and washing the patients. Obviously she was hoping that someone else would deal

The mistakes continue

with Charlie before she got there, so she wouldn't have to. The lunch trolley arrived and finally one of the nurses came over to see to Charlie. "Come on, I'm here to change you now," she said, then stripped and washed him and the bed. It was 12:13 pm. They gave Charlie his meal, but he refused to eat anything. I went over to talk to him after lunch and asked him why he hadn't eaten. I felt awful about all that had happened and I didn't want him to start getting even weaker. He looked at me and said, "if I don't eat, then I won't have to lie in my own mess."

I was so disgusted by that nurse that I reported her to the director for nursing, who in turn reported her to the staff nurse on duty that shift. The staff nurse came into Paul's room and started crying, she was so embarrassed about what had been done to poor Charlie. I had started documenting the care that was given to the elderly patients shortly after Paul was admitted to the ward. It had become apparent to us fairly early on that he would be in hospital for some time, as no one could find out what was wrong with him and his condition was too delicate for intensive tests. I was there all day every day and often had time on my hands, so I began to take notes. As well as patients being left lying for hours in their own excrement, I noted how widespread the problem of dehydration was. I watched the way the nurses filled out the fluid charts. They couldn't usually see me from where I sat in Paul's room, but I had a pretty good view of a lot of them. The nurses would go around filling out the charts and sometimes the patients would be asleep so the nurses would just take a guess at what they had taken, maybe assuming that they had drunk their morning juice and tea, but never really knowing for sure. Even if the patient wasn't asleep when the nurses came around to fill in their charts, half of them couldn't remember how much water they had drunk that day, so the nurses would guess. I knew that many nurses were not aware of the potential harm they were causing their patients by doing this and I suppose that was the main reason that I began to document everything. A normal, healthy person will drink when they feel thirsty and in this way the body regulates itself by letting you know what it needs. But an elderly person is not always aware of what

The mistakes continue

they need and once they begin to dehydrate, then they get even more confused and rapidly deteriorate. Even when they do feel thirsty, they sometimes cannot reach their water, or maybe they don't have any left and they don't usually like to ask for things for fear of being thought a nuisance. I remember that one of the nurses took two days off once and on her return was checking through some patients' charts. I heard her ask the other nurses, "why hasn't anyone filled in the patients' food and water charts in the two days I've been off?"

Someone else called back, "sorry, we just didn't have enough time."

"Well, I suppose I'll just have to do it myself then," she responded.

I was horrified. What makes all this even worse is that while most nurses do not properly monitor fluid and food intake, they do stick to a fairly accurate timetable for medication. So while these patients were being given their pills every four hours, no one was making sure that they drank enough water to live. Now that Paul had his electric chair, he seemed to be on a mission to make sure that people drank the proper amount of water. He would zip around from bed to bed, pour the person a glass of water and then sit there while they drank it. When they were done, he would refill the glass and then put it within easy reach of the patient. He would stress the importance of drinking water to them and just sit there and chat with each one of them for a few minutes. I was so proud of him. I can't help but feel that he did as much for some of those patients as the doctors and nurses did.

I remember one gentleman who got quite ill and had nothing to eat or drink for two days. The nurses never mentioned it to his visiting relatives, maybe because they were afraid the family members would think they weren't taking good care of the man. Or maybe the nurses hadn't even noticed. Many mornings the man would wake up confused and everyone just put it down to his age. But that wasn't the case. It was obvious to me that he was dehydrating and then being pumped full of drugs on top of that. Several times, I wanted to go over and mention something to his

The mistakes continue

daughter. I thought that at least if she was aware of it, she could sit and encourage him to sip some water or maybe bring in bits of his favourite foods. But I just couldn't bring myself to make a scene.

I know that nurses don't usually like family members taking too big a role in caring for patients and I could never understand that. They were constantly complaining about how short-staffed they were. I would have thought that we were doing them a favour. But whether they liked it or not, I was always going to be there for Paul, because it was quite clear to me that this was the only way he would be properly cared for. Seeing what happened to Charlie and others like him made Paul even more determined that I wasn't to leave him. To this day, I live with the guilt that maybe I realised too late that he needed me to protect him. That maybe if I had been more attentive earlier on, I could have prevented a lot of his injuries. But then I think, 'why should I have been the one looking after his medical needs when he was in hospital surrounded by doctors and nurses and I had no medical training at all?'

As time went on, I watched Paul become more and more emotionally distressed and though I tried to alleviate it, in truth I could see how justified it was. Patients are allowed so little dignity in hospital and are given so little support outside of it. I didn't even want to think about how he would have been treated if I hadn't been there all the time. It scared me to think that perhaps he was right in not wanting to live anymore.

It was early August and Paul had been in the hospital for about seven weeks. They still hadn't established what was wrong with him, though they were pretty sure that gallstones were at least one of the problems. An appointment had been booked with a new surgeon, but not until September. Paul wasn't in any sort of condition to do some of the more exploratory investigations and, since he wasn't getting any worse, they decided that he could go home and they would wait to see what happened. Every other time he had been released from hospital, I had been anxious to get him home, but this time was a little different. Of course we were all happy to have him back, but I was nervous as well. I had trained

The mistakes continue

for all of his physical problems and I could handle those, but I wasn't so sure about his mental state. He was so sad all of the time and I just didn't know what to do about it. I kept praying that someone would help and that they wouldn't leave everything up to me.

On the day he was released, Adam and Lee got a van again, so that they could bring home his chair. Sheba went mad when he came into the house; she had been missing him so much. Sheba became Paul's guardian when he was home and would patrol the fences and the front window, then go back to Paul and sniff him to make sure he was OK. Paul had a box of doggy sweets by the side of his chair and he would feed them to her all day long. He loved her to pieces and spoiled her. It was lovely to see him happy for a bit, but she was one of his few pleasures. We settled back into a routine at home, but things were definitely different this time. There was a look about Paul's face. I had seen him look sad before, but this was permanent.

My mum came around one day with some photos she had taken a couple of months before. We had gone to visit her and I was walking up to her house, pushing Paul in his wheelchair. It was early June, the sun was shining and it was a beautiful day. I remembered her asking us to wait while she took some pictures. She had copies made so that we could keep them. I looked at the photos and I could actually see that Paul hadn't wanted to be there. Not there at my mum's, but there at all. How could I have missed it at the time? I suppose I just hadn't wanted to see it. But in addition to the sadness, there were other emotions on his face as well. There was fear and torment. It confused me – did he want to die or didn't he? It must have confused him as well.

One day soon after his release, Paul and I planned to go over to the supermarket for some lunch and then to do our shopping there. His bowels were still bothering him, but if we timed things right, then he could manage to enjoy himself a bit. He loved getting out of the house anyway. When we got to the café portion of the supermarket, I took Paul over to the food counter so that he could see what was being offered and decide what he wanted. Once he had made up his mind, I took him over to a table and got him settled, then went back to order the food. I brought all the condiments and utensils over to our table and we waited for the food to be delivered.

Paul looked at me then and mouthed, "I don't have a choice, do I?"

"About what?" I asked.

"About staying alive."

"Don't be silly, everyone has choices."

"Well, I don't have any." I could tell he was beginning to get angry. "There are things going wrong with me now because of the negligence and the doctors are afraid to treat me. If they would pay my compensation, then I could go private and get myself sorted out. But that's not going to happen yet. Even if social services would help us, then maybe we could get through, but I have thought about it and I don't have any choice but to end it. I'm scared of choking to death or of the pain coming back and knowing that no one will help me. I can't live with this fear anymore." There were tears in his eyes and I could feel them building in mine as well.

"I'll never let you choke to death Paul, I promise. If the pain comes back, we have some tablets of MST at home that will take care of it."

He looked at me fondly and mouthed, "you always have an answer don't you? Still full of optimism. Well, I haven't any hope anymore, don't you understand that? I want to be in control of my own death, not them. They have done enough to me without taking that away from me too. If I left it to them, I would probably die in tremendous pain or very scared and choking in a hospital ward."

It was my turn to get cross then and I said to him, "it'll never be left to them, you know that! I have always been there for you and always will."

"But what happens if something happens to you?"

"We will face that when and if it happens."

"No," he insisted, "I am not leaving my death to chance."

The mistakes continue

Our food came just then and we both sat staring at it, our tempers frayed and our eyes watery. Paul began again, "please understand me, I have to do this because I don't have any other choice, I don't want to live this way anymore."

"I understand the way you feel, but what about me? What will I do when you're gone?"

"You'll go on. You have Adam and Lee and you'll meet someone else. You're still young and you deserve to have a better life than this, spending all your time caring for an invalid. You'll be OK, I promise." I was about to protest, to tell him that I never resented having to care for him and that I wouldn't have it any other way, but he wasn't finished yet. He started asking me about compensation and how his death would affect the amount that we got, particularly if he took his own life. I told him that I had no idea and he asked me to ask our lawyer. I agreed, but couldn't imagine how to broach the topic with her. Then I thought of something else. "How do you plan to take your life?" I asked him, swallowing the lump in my throat and wondering just how we had reached the point where my husband's suicide options were the sort of conversation that we had over lunch. The tears were rolling down my face by now. He looked at me, smiled and simply mouthed, "let's eat up, get the shopping and then go home." As we were driving home, Paul turned to me and mouthed, "I have thought about ways to do it, but I'd rather not tell you. That way you won't stop me and you won't know when I'm going to do it."

Now Paul wanted to get everything written down and sorted out and make sure everything was as legal as it could be. It was important to him that I speak to the lawyer and find out how his death would affect the rest of us legally and financially. He assured me that he didn't plan to do it immediately and, though he didn't state it specifically, it was obvious he intended to wait at least until this was all settled.

That evening after dinner, Adam and Lee went to football training and we turned off the TV and sat down to talk. I let Paul do most of the talking, as it was obvious that there were so many things he needed to say. It was difficult to follow him some of the

The mistakes continue

time, as he would often get emotional and then hang his head down. I was forced to ask him to look up, interrupting him in the middle of him telling me his most personal thoughts to repeat himself. That just reminded him even more of how much his body had been mutilated and how much he wanted to go back to the way things were. "I've thought about how I will take my own life and I'm happy enough that it will work. I'm a bit scared that I will have a heart attack as a result of what I'm going to do, but at least I won't choke to death. I'm sorry things haven't been better for us," he began to mouth, but I couldn't help jumping in at that point.

"We had a wonderful marriage, you know that!" I insisted and it was true. "We've had our ups and downs, but that's the same in every marriage." I was crying now and just couldn't bear him thinking that he was to blame for anything when he was in the state that he was in. I didn't want him finding fault with himself when he was already so depressed that he didn't think his life was worth living.

"I wish I had been a better husband to you…" he tried to continue, but I just couldn't cope with the way this conversation was going. I tried to make him feel better, but it seemed to have no effect. He continued on in the same vein, saying that he didn't feel he had been a good father to Adam and Lee either. It was then that I told him this had to stop. He had been a wonderful father and the proof was that we had two wonderful boys.

I looked into his eyes and knew that I could never leave him alone again, not even for a second. If he had to go back to hospital, then the three of us would take turns and would stay overnight in his room and sleep in a chair. I didn't want him to ever be afraid again and felt so guilty for having left him before. What I wanted most of all then was for the conversation to be over, it was so painful for me to see my husband so afraid and not to be able to do anything about it.

Chapter 13

Hoping for help

I called our lawyer up a few days later and discussed the issues that Paul had been so eager to clear up. The first had to do with getting independent doctors to confirm that his illnesses had been caused by negligence. She was tracking down experts in various fields, but it was hard to get Paul around the country. Still she was working on it and I had the utmost confidence that it would get done. I then broached the subject of Paul's death and how it would affect our claim. She informed me that it would still be paid into Paul's estate, but that the amount we received would be substantially reduced. I asked her why that was and received a mini crash-course in negligence law. The amount of Paul's claim was based on two things, personal damage and future care. The first was to compensate him for the pain and suffering he had been made to endure at the hands of the NHS. The second was for the care that would be required for him until he died and began from the time of his first being dehydrated. As it had only been a couple of years since he had been neglected by the NHS, then the bulk of his claim lay in his future care. If he were to die, then there would no longer be any need for them to give us this money.

I found the logic of the legal system terribly wrong. A person is made very ill by the hospitals and needs extra care and special facilities in their homes to have a basic standard of living. This requires money, so they file a claim. The legal system then makes the victim wait so long while they drag out the proceedings, that they become completely miserable from lack of funds and eventually get to the point where they want to end their lives. Then the legal system reduces the payment substantially because the abused person is no longer alive and does not need to be taken care of. In other words, the longer the legal system dragged things out, the less they would have to pay, especially if the patient got so desperate that he killed himself. Paul and I sat down to discuss what I had spoken to our lawyer about and Paul summed it up neatly. "So, if I stay alive, we will probably get about one million pounds, then I could kill myself. But if I kill myself now, then you will get next to nothing in compensation. So, if I kill myself, then I am actually saving the NHS a lot of money." I had never wanted money to be a factor in his decision to end his own life, but if it would keep him alive a bit longer, then was it so bad? Paul's family had never been rich and to people who grow up with no money, it becomes a very important thing. I knew he hated the idea that I and the boys would have to struggle for money because of his illnesses. Perhaps, if he waited a bit, then we would get the money and I could use it to make his life better and then he would want to stay with us. "Yes, that's what it seems to be," I said to him.

The detective called me a few days later to tell me that he wanted to stop by our house and update us on his investigation. We arranged a meeting in several days time, but when he came over, his expression was pretty glum. Firstly, he explained, there were no grounds for charging the chief executive with anything criminal. Secondly, he claimed that they could not ascertain whose signature it was on Paul's discharge plan for 27th September. He still thought that it was quite likely that of a junior doctor who had returned to South Africa, but he hadn't been able to track him down. Finally, the blood test results from 27th September, which revealed that Paul had been released in full renal failure, were now back in his medical records so now, two years after the event, there was no way to prove that they had ever been removed or by whom. He would leave the case open, he told me, in case anything else was found out, but for now his investigation was finished. He then gave me the standard answer that everyone seemed to be giving me in those days, "at least the NHS have admitted liability."

Hoping for help

I was sickened that nothing had come out of the police investigation. After all, I had provided evidence to the police that the chief executive had received a copy of the 27th September blood test results about a week before he wrote a letter to me claiming that the last blood tests had been done on Paul on the 26th September. Moreover, I had told the police precisely which doctor had signed Paul's discharge form and that the doctor was in Birmingham and not in South Africa as the NHS seemed to be suggesting. Yet it appeared as if all the documents I had produced had been ignored and that the police were accepting the NHS's version of events. I was sure that several individuals had committed crimes against Paul. But what really worried me now was how Paul would handle the disappointing outcome of the police's work. I could see him looking down at his stumps and I knew he couldn't believe that no one was going to be held accountable for all the damage that had been done to him. I felt physically ill. As I looked at Paul, I knew there was no way that I could ever let this rest. Even if it didn't directly benefit us, hopefully it would help someone somewhere at some time. I knew that we were not unique and there must be many others who had things suddenly "disappear" from their files. I couldn't understand how someone could look at a person who had been injured as much as Paul had and care more about protecting their own careers than about trying to care for him and taking responsibility for what had gone wrong. Everybody makes mistakes, even doctors, so why not come to terms with it and try to make the victim's life a little bit more liveable? What made me even angrier was that these same people were probably at the height of their careers and well-respected and well-paid. Whereas people like us, people whom they had wronged, were left to scrape by as best we could. Perhaps the police couldn't or didn't want to bring them to justice, but I would certainly carry on the fight.

Paul began to get really nasty over the next few weeks and it seemed as if there was nothing that I could do right. He would pick on Adam and Lee as well and seemed to be doing everything in his power to start fights. We tried to ignore him as best we could and deal with his abuse, because he was obviously depressed. But I think part of me stopped coping then and stopped caring on a certain level, because I just couldn't deal with all that was happening anymore. I knew that it would be relatively easy for him to kill himself, he could just take too much medication or insulin and every day I wondered if today would be the day. The man I have been living with for so many years was going to kill himself and I had no idea how I would cope on my own. We were both having nightmares by this point and I had lost six stone.

I was still trying to take him out every day, even if only for a drive. Some days he didn't want to go out at all because he was tired of people staring at him and I was usually too fed up to argue. On one particular day, we decided to go to Coventry town centre. Paul usually loved being pushed around the town centre and we had a routine that we liked to follow. First we could go to M&S and walk around the food hall, picking up little goodies that he felt like having. Then we would go to our favourite butcher's at the other end of town where he would get some pies and cooked meat for the boys to have later. He had begun paying some money into a club earlier that year to save for Christmas, so if we had a bit extra we would put some in while we were there. After that we would go back to the centre and get Paul a fresh baguette to eat while we sat around the fountain. On this particular occasion we did things a bit differently and decided that we would have a meal out. Near the butcher's was a trendy little café that we had passed by several times and Paul had mentioned once that it looked lovely, but he didn't think that he would ever be able to get his wheelchair in there. I thought it would be a nice treat for him that day, so I went in to have a look and see whether or not it would be possible.

As it turned out, the seats were fixed to the floor and the tables were very close together, so it was obvious to me that it wouldn't work. I turned to go, quite disappointed and then noticed that there was a table right near the door that had moveable chairs and the people that had been sitting there were just getting up to leave. It seemed a stroke of luck, so I put my shopping down at the

Hoping for help

table and went outside to get Paul. It took some manoeuvring to get him into the space I had made for him by moving a couple of chairs. I had to weave his chair in between a couple of tables to get him in there and of course by now we had attracted some attention. I sat down opposite him, a bit flustered and out of breath and could see that he was really cross. I suppose I should have known better than to try to get him into a café that was so tightly packed, but I had only done it to try and cheer him up. People were looking at us and he felt as if I had made an exhibition of him. After I had ordered food for us, he didn't want to talk to me, so we just sat there in silence eating our dinners. I looked out the window and saw people hurrying all over the place doing their shopping and getting on with their business and remembered the days when Paul and I used to do things like that. My eyes filled up with tears, I just couldn't help it.

Paul leaned forward and mouthed, "what are you trying to do now, make even more people look at us?" I just turned away and tried to get my emotions under control. All of a sudden he started banging on the table so loudly that everybody turned to look at us. "Take me home right now!" he ordered me. I stood up. I was so embarrassed, I didn't know what else to do. People just smiled at me and carried on eating. I'm sure they thought that I was having a day out with a mentally disabled person. I got Paul out of there as quickly as I could and practically ran with him to the car. I made him get into the car on his own and we didn't speak a word to one another for the rest of that day. I watched him that night as he sat in his chair, totally absorbed in his own thoughts with a tormented look on his face. I was scared, as always, that tonight might be the night he killed himself. But I also thought to myself, 'you are not the only one who's tormented.'

An appointment had finally come through for a barium enema X-ray for Paul. There is a certain amount of preparation that has to be done before this, so I went over the details quite carefully. The procedure is different for someone with diabetes than it is for others and as I was reading the instructions, I saw that they were not intended for a diabetic. I was furious. After all that had happened, I couldn't believe that a doctor would be careless enough not to read Paul's file beforehand and know that he was diabetic. It was plastered all over his medical records, not to mention that he was so obviously a special-needs person, that extra care should be taken before prescribing any treatment for him at all. Obviously the letter that the hospital had inserted into the front of his file, warning doctors to read his records carefully, had no effect. Paul was flabbergasted that they could still get things wrong for him and still possibly even do him more damage.

I marched over to the hospital on Monday morning and went to the X-ray department, demanding an explanation. They confirmed that the wrong test had been ordered for Paul and issued a new one straight away. I wrote to the director of nursing that very night to complain and to ask how it was possible that mistakes were still being made about Paul's treatment. She skirted around me for a while, but eventually got around to writing me an apology letter the following year. She missed the point entirely of course, I didn't want apology letters, I wanted medical professionals who would care for my husband properly. It obviously didn't matter much to them, but I wanted him to stay alive. Though for them, it would certainly be a lot cheaper and more convenient if he died.

Paul decided that he didn't want to go in for the X-ray anyway, as he didn't see that it would do him any good. He was sick of them getting things wrong and most of the time seeming to do him more harm than good. It took some persuasion, but eventually I did change his mind and got him to let me take him over there. As we were leaving the hospital after the appointment, he mouthed to me, "I don't want to go back there ever again, there's no point." Unfortunately, I could see only too well why he would think so, but I wanted to encourage him to try to get better. I didn't want to disagree with him and make him angry, so I just said, "well let's see as we go along."

"You can't make me go," he mouthed to me, with a stubborn look on his face.

Hoping for help

"I know I can't and I wouldn't try to make you anyway, but I just thought that maybe this feeling is a phase because the hospital has let you down again. Maybe things will get better later on and you'll feel differently." My words sounded hollow even to me and I knew that this would be just more proof to Paul that he could not leave the circumstances of his death to the hospital.

By now our suicide discussions had reached the point where we talked often about what Paul wished for after his death, what he wanted for his sons and for me. We broke down in tears just about every time we talked about Adam's and Lee's futures. Paul wanted so desperately to be a part of it and of course I wanted him there too. We talked on occasions about what Paul believed would happen to him after he died and I'm certain that the out-of-body experience that he believed he had on the night of 29th September when he went into a coma made his decision to take his own life easier. He felt that the same grey-haired old man would most likely be waiting for him when he died, even though he didn't actually know who the man was. He thought of him as a sort of guide, one that would lead him to his parents.

I had always known that he wanted to be cremated, but we had only recently discussed what he wanted done with his ashes afterwards. He sometimes thought he would like to have them buried next to his mum and dad, but at other times he didn't seem to think that it would matter at all, since he wouldn't be aware of it. In the end he told me to just do whatever I thought was appropriate and that he would be happy with whatever I chose. Thoughts of his parents would lead us to reminisce about the days when they had been alive. He still missed his mum terribly, though she had been dead about fifteen months by that point. Mainly we would remember what a wonderful sense of humour she had and how she would laugh and laugh for minutes on end when she found something funny. She would have to keep her legs tightly crossed at those times because she was laughing so hard she feared she might wet herself. She would set the rest of us going, even if we didn't necessarily know what it was we were laughing about.

Hoping for help

One morning in September, Paul woke up in a foul mood. He wouldn't eat his porridge and went ahead and injected his own insulin without waiting for me to help. He used an insulin pen and though he could draw the insulin into the pen on his own, he did not have the strength in his fingers to pump it out. That morning he was so angry with the world that he just jabbed the needle into his stomach and roughly pressed down on the end of it to get all the insulin out. I went over to him, saying, "what are you doing? Give it to me and let me help you." He pushed me away and swore at me, telling me to leave him alone. I wasn't sure how to deal with him in this mood, so I just went into the kitchen to finish the washing up. I hoped that if I gave him a bit of time, he would calm down and then we could get on with the day. I felt completely out of my depth. I had called social services in June and July and still no one had come back to me. I had told all of Paul's doctors and our solicitor about his frame of mind, but no one seemed to be able or willing to help us. I didn't know how much longer I could go on as we were, but I just tried to take things one day at a time and hope that Paul would still be alive at the end of it. When I had finished the washing up, I went into the lounge where Paul was watching TV. "Do you want to get showered now," I asked him, my stomach a flurry of nerves as I waited for whatever fresh abuse he might choose to throw my way. But all he said was "yes" and I felt relieved that he had calmed down a bit. Perhaps the day could be salvaged after all.

I showered him, changed his tracky dressings and massaged his stump, then began helping him to put his clothes on. "Do you want to into town today?" I asked, hoping to brighten his mood. "No, why don't you go on your own," he answered. I just looked at him, wondering if this was his idea of a joke. He knew perfectly well that I would never leave him alone in the house. Even if Adam or Lee had been there, I wouldn't leave them alone with him when he was in that sort of mood. Besides which, I was only suggesting that we go out to get him out of the house as there was nothing that I needed to do in town. But I didn't want to start an argument with him, so I just nodded and didn't say anything. I

196

Hoping for help

went into the kitchen to do some more tidying. Paul came to the kitchen door a few minutes later. "I've been thinking," he mouthed, "why don't you, Adam and Lee try to find a flat and start a new life?"

"What's wrong with you?" I asked angrily, having had about enough of his attitude for one day. "Why are you doing this?"

"I don't love you anymore," he blurted out.

I was devastated. We had had many arguments over the years and called each other some pretty cruel names, but neither one of us had ever said anything like that. We had always known, no matter what we were fighting about, that our marriage was still based on love. I still loved him and, after all that I had done for him, I didn't understand how he could say that to me. I dried my hands and sat down, my eyes filling with tears. I spent most of the rest of the day crying – every time I thought I was finished, I would hear his words in my head and it would start all over again. Paul stayed out of my way for the rest of the day, sulking in his chair for hours. When Adam and Lee came home from work that evening, they knew that something was wrong. Right away, Adam asked me, "what's wrong?"

Just as quickly I responded, "your dad told me today that he doesn't love me anymore and wants us to move out of the house."

Both of them immediately said, "of course he doesn't mean that mum."

"He shouldn't have said it then," I replied, feeling the tears begin to fill my eyes again.

The boys generally tried to stay out of Paul's way when he was in a bad mood, as I did. Unfortunately Paul's bad moods were happening more and more often these days. But I suppose the sight of me in tears was more than either of them could take because they both went over and stood in front of his chair. "Why have you said that to mum, dad? She is the only person who has fought and cared for you through all of this," Adam said. Paul for once didn't know how to answer. He just sat and looked at his hands. "You had better apologise to mum and put it right." Still Paul did nothing. Adam, seeing he wasn't getting anywhere with Paul, came back over to me and repeated, "he didn't mean it mum." I wasn't so sure. After so many years of knowing everything that needed to be known about Paul, I found that I couldn't understand what he was feeling when he got into these dark moods. Perhaps he thought I should be doing more for him? Maybe he thought that I hadn't been forceful enough in seeing to his needs in hospital? Or did he just blame me for taking him back to the hospital so many times, instead of letting him die? Either way, I knew that I couldn't do any more for him than I had done and didn't think I could continue on much longer the way things were going between us.

I knew that we needed to start spending some time apart. I almost never left his side and it was beginning to wear on both of us. I blamed social services for much of this, because they had never got back to us about organising carers for Paul or perhaps group sessions that he could go to without me, where he would be properly looked after by trained medics. We both needed to get our lives back, altered though they were. Adam had been talking about joining a gym up in Bedworth to try to lose some weight and it seemed like the perfect opportunity for me to get out of the house. I had lost a lot of weight already, but still had a fair way to go and desperately needed a change of scenery. I decided that I would discuss it with Adam and Lee the next day, as it would mean them being there to look after Paul. That night I cared for Paul in silence, changing his dressings and helping him out of his clothes. When he got me angry, I sometimes wanted to make things tough for him, but I had never and would never leave him to do something I knew he was incapable of. He accepted my help without a word and went to sleep without apologising to me.

The following morning, I called our lawyer to ask her about a consultant that we needed to make an appointment with to discuss Paul's case. We chatted about legal things for a while, but I was still so upset that I ended up breaking down and telling her what Paul had said to me the day before. Paul was in the room, but just continued to ignore me and watch TV. "Calm down," the

Hoping for help

lawyer told me, "let's just think for a moment and analyse what he said. We both know that he has been depressed lately and thinking about suicide. If you ask me, I think he is just trying to create some distance between the two of you, to make taking his life that much easier. Not only for him, but for you as well. Maybe he thinks that if he makes you angry with him, you will stop loving him so much and then won't miss him so much when he's gone. If it makes you feel any better, I have a lot of respect for you and I have no idea how you manage to cope. I really admire your strength and determination – I don't know if I would have been able to handle things as well as you have."

I thought about what she said and had to admit that it made sense to me. It was still wrong of Paul to say what he had said, but at least now I could understand what had made him say it. As long as I was able to believe that he didn't mean it, it made it a lot easier to deal with. We went back to speaking about social services and our claim against the hospital, which I found easier to concentrate on now that she had soothed me about what Paul had said. She was quite angry that social services still had not been in contact with us after so many months. She told me that she was doing her best to hurry things up at her end. The thought of getting a bit of money to ease the situation gave me new hope. I would do my best to keep Paul alive until then and try not to take his abuse too personally. By the time we ended the phone call, I was feeling a bit more like myself.

Paul gave no indication that he had heard our phone conversation and still did not apologise to me for his words of the day before. He did treat me quite gently that morning though, which made me believe that he was sorry. He wanted to go out, so I began to get him ready. He had been having some circulation problems with his stump recently, which was very worrying. Sometimes when they do a below-the-knee amputation, it doesn't heal properly for one reason or another and then they have to go back and remove more of the leg. If we didn't want the entire leg to be removed, we had to take special care of what was left - that included Paul keeping the stump elevated at every opportunity.

Hoping for help

Normally this was not difficult, as Paul's remote-controlled chair was reclining and we had a board that fitted onto the frame of his wheelchair. I had to massage the stump quite often, trying to improve the circulation, but it was still a blue-black colour. Not that it really mattered, practically speaking, whether Paul's leg was cut off above or below the knee, but I didn't want him to have to undergo yet another operation. The chances of him surviving it, provided that we could find a doctor willing to perform it and that I could convince Paul himself that it was worth doing, were very slim indeed.

My dad's sister, Joyce, had a son named Allan who ran a bookshop in the town centre. Ever since I could remember, he had been involved in local councils and politics and though I didn't know what, if anything, I expected him to be able to do for us, I thought it wouldn't hurt to talk to him. I was so frustrated at being ignored by social services and with the hospital dragging their feet on our compensation claim, that I was willing to talk to just about anyone. So the following week, I decided to pay him a visit at his shop. Paul didn't think it would be worthwhile talking to him, but he did want to go for a little outing, so he accompanied me to town. It was a Wednesday, which was market day, so we bought some fresh fruit, then went to get some toffee from Thornton's. By then Paul was hungry – not unusual as it took so much time and effort to get him ready that by the time we got anywhere it was usually lunchtime. We went to a nearby café, which was one of the only places that he still felt comfortable going. Most of the staff there remembered him from the days when he could walk and it was spacious without fixed seats, so it was easy to manoeuvre his wheelchair around. We came here often, so no one stared at Paul anymore and the waitresses even knew how to read his lips and take his food order directly from him. We often saw people we knew there, as it was a regular haunt for hospital staff.

After lunch, we headed over to the bookshop, which was at the other end of town. As we got near, Paul turned around in his chair and asked me not to take him into the store. "Why?" I asked, surprised. "I just hate watching you tell our whole story all over again and getting so upset and crying. I hate having to see you resort to begging, so please just leave me outside." There was a little alley at the side of the shop and Paul asked me to park his chair there and not to keep him waiting too long. I thought I would be able to see him from inside the shop, so didn't see the harm in it. I still wasn't sure what I was expecting Allan to do, as he belonged to the opposite political party from our MP, who had been helping us so far, but at the very least it would give me a chance to talk to someone.

I told him our story and like everybody else, he seemed astounded at first, then indignant, then horrified. Of course he had known some of it already through the family, but he didn't know anything about my attempts to get help from social services and the fact that they had been ignoring us. He told me that he was involved with the Warwickshire County Council and asked if I wanted him to speak to someone on my behalf and try to get someone to pay attention to us. I thanked him, but tried to remind myself not to get my hopes up. Not that I didn't think he would try to help us, but felt we had just got nowhere despite all my efforts. On the way to the car, I told Paul what we had spoken about, but he just shrugged. He had gone beyond the point of caring by then. Our MP also came by to see us the following weekend and was equally upset that social services had still not been around to see us. He told me that he would be in touch with the chief executive and would do his best to get them moving on our case.

It was now almost two years since the hospital had discharged Paul in renal failure. It didn't look to either of us as if there was an end in sight for our claim. So when our lawyer called to say that the NHS lawyers wanted a meeting, we were overjoyed. It was to be a meeting 'without prejudice' (this meant they were not committed to anything they said in the meeting) and our lawyer had agreed for it to take place at her office the following Wednesday. She thought that they might make an offer there and then, but warned us that they normally made a very low initial offer and that it would take time to negotiate with them for something more reasonable.

We had also received the initial assessment from the care company, which stated that Paul would need five people to care for him full-time and that the estimated cost of this was £180,000 a year. A more in-depth assessment would have to be done later on, but this was certainly sufficient for our lawyer to approach the NHS lawyers with a request for some kind of payment. They would never pay that amount, of course, and would bargain us down, but at least we would hopefully get some help.

Meanwhile, I was still receiving anonymous pamphlets and letters from the nurse who had sent us the letter with copies of Paul's 'missing' blood test results and whom I had begun to think of as our guardian angel at the hospital. The particular set of papers I received around that time had to do with the removal of Paul's blood test results from his file. The police had decided that they didn't have enough evidence to prosecute anyone and had stopped investigating, but the issue was still very much alive in our minds. The apparent reluctance of both the police and the hospital to discover who had removed the results made me suspect that it must be someone very high up. The envelope that we now received contained a memo from the medical filing office confirming that Paul Steane's medical records had been brought up to date at the chief executive's request and that the 27th September blood test results (which proved Paul had been discharged in renal failure) had been reprinted and inserted. This had all happened on the 22nd and 23rd March, about a week before our meeting with the chief executive at which he had claimed the last blood tests done on Paul had been on 26th September. Also included was a schedule of meetings that the hospital chief executive was to attend to discuss our claim against the hospital and a note saying "Good luck." I was left to contemplate the meaning of these documents on my own, as Paul was no longer bothered. To be honest, I wasn't sure if I was either. I had reached the point where I had begun to just want to be out of the situation in any way possible. I didn't feel that way all the time, but it scared me when I did. I was no longer just worried about Paul's frame of mind, but my own as well.

One day I opened the drawer beside Paul's bed and noticed that there were MST pills in there. I picked up the packet, which was full, and counted twenty six of them. I was suspicious, as these were very dangerous tablets. I went back into the lounge straight away to ask Paul about them. "Oh, they've been there since I had all that stomach pain in June," he quickly replied. "I took them out of the medication drawer just in case it came back and I needed them quickly. Besides, I didn't want them in the family drawer in case Adam or Lee accidentally took them one day when they weren't paying attention. I thought they would be safer in my own drawer." I agreed with that, so I tried to ignore the feeling in my stomach that something wasn't right. I hated having such dangerous drugs in the house at all, but I knew that it was very possible that Paul might need them again at some point. So I put them back.

Paul sunk deeper and deeper into his depression, convinced that if we finally did receive compensation, he would be too ill to be able to enjoy it. He pulled me down with him and I was finding it increasingly difficult to go on taking care of him when I got no thanks for it and when he was so often abusive. I understood how desperate he felt, but it didn't make it any easier to deal with when he was taking most of it out on me. Adam and Lee picked up on the difficulties that we were having and tried to pitch in a little bit more in caring for Paul. Adam had begun taking him to football games at Coventry City, knowing how much his dad loved watching them play. It was very hard for him to get Paul around and at first he was very nervous that Paul would need some sort of medical treatment while they were out, that he wouldn't be able to provide. But he wanted to do something for his father and for me as well. By now both he and Lee were quite adept at taking care of Paul, but I always had my mobile with me in case of an emergency.

I had decided that I would join the gym after all, to keep my sanity. I would go for an hour every night, except for Sundays,

Hoping for help

leaving Lee to care for Paul most of the time, though sometimes Adam did it when Lee couldn't. I absolutely loved having time to myself, just walking on the treadmill with loud music blasting in my ears and letting my mind wander. I could pretend that my life wasn't what it was and would leave there feeling refreshed. Sometimes, if I had a bad day with Paul, I couldn't even bring myself to enter the gym. Then I would sit in the car, talking to friends on my mobile. Or I would just drive around, with the music blasting to distract me. Either way, I would end up shedding lots of tears. But at least it got me out of the house for a bit. There were times when I just wanted to run away, never see Paul again and never change another dressing or massage another stump. He would make me feel so unloved and used when he got into his moods. I tried to push these thoughts away, but I had to admit to myself that they were becoming more and more frequent.

On the night of the 4th October, I arrived back from the gym to find Paul in good spirits. I wouldn't realise it for several months, but that night he would try to commit suicide for the first time. We had bought a fresh baguette from the baker's and he asked me to make him a ham and tomato sandwich with some crisps and a cup of tea. I was pleased to see him in such a good mood, so I went straight into the kitchen to get started. Paul got himself into his electric chair and came to watch me from the kitchen door. I started telling him how nice it would be if he could come to the gym with me sometime. "There's a lift," I said, trying to tempt him, "so it would be easy for you to get in." He had been doing some upper body exercises at home with dumbbells that we had bought, as well as deep breathing exercises twice a day. I told him that he could continue to do that at the gym and be able to work his muscles more effectively. But he was too self-conscious. "I'm too embarrassed to go to a gym with the way I look," he mouthed, shaking his head.

That night we went to bed as normal and I dropped off quite quickly. I was physically tired from the gym, but more than that, I was emotionally drained. Even though that day had been a good one, it was the daily grind that was wearing me down, the

Hoping for help

constant pressure of having to take care of Paul and never knowing when he would finally decide to take that last step. At some point in the night, I became aware that Paul was very restless and I was half-awake when I thought I saw him going into the lounge to watch TV. It was rare, but sometimes Paul would do that if he couldn't sleep and didn't want to disturb me. But it must have just melted into whatever dream I was having, because I drifted off again. The next morning was Saturday and I woke up to find that Paul wasn't in bed with me. I shot up, looked at the clock and saw that I had overslept. My heart began to pound, but then I realised that Paul was breathing so loudly that I could hear him all the way from the lounge. I thought he might be having problems because of his granulation, so I got dressed quickly and went to see if I could help.

The back of Paul's chair was facing the lounge entrance, but as I entered I could see his arm hanging down the side, limp. Scared, I rushed around to the front of the chair and he was just slumped there, eyes open, but not conscious. He couldn't see or hear me and I didn't dare touch him. I ran to the door and screamed for Adam and Lee to come downstairs. They couldn't have been too deeply asleep, because they got there quite quickly. Adam stood in front of Paul, trying to talk to him, while I went to call the ambulance. None of us wanted to move him until we knew what was going on. I was shaking, thinking that he must have had a stroke, which had been another one of his fears. He had already lost the ability to walk and talk, but losing the ability to move at all would be the absolute end for Paul.

I went back to stand in front of Paul while we waited for the ambulance to arrive, thinking that if he had suffered a stroke, maybe he could still see and hear us, even if he couldn't respond. I kept talking to him and thought that I saw his eyelids flicker slightly, but I couldn't be certain. I felt faint and was worried that I would pass out and then the medics would have me to deal with as well. Soon we could hear the ambulance in the distance, so I sent Adam out to open the front door for them. As he was turning to go, he said to me, "you know mum, this might be dad's diabetes."

205

Hoping for help

"I don't know Adam. I don't think so." Paul had never gone into a diabetic coma before and he had had the disease for many years now. His blood sugar had gone very low on many occasions, but he had never lost consciousness. Adam seemed convinced though and I found myself hoping that he was right. That would be something easily fixable.

When the medics came into the lounge, they immediately began taking out heart monitors and blood pressure instruments. One of them began speaking to Paul, trying to get a response. Adam said to them, "it might be dad's diabetes."

One of them looked at me and asked, "is he diabetic?"

"Yes," I responded, "insulin dependent."

They pricked his finger to check his blood-sugar level and found that it was at one – dangerously low. We were all relieved that the problem had been identified so quickly. They began looking for a vein in Paul's arm in which to insert a needle, but seemed to be having difficulty. I told them that most doctors did because of his having been kept on life-support for so long. The noradrenalin that had been pumped into him to keep him alive was a vascular constrictor and many of his veins had contracted. I ran to fetch the glucose tablets that I kept for emergencies and gave them to the paramedics. They placed one under Paul's tongue and waited for it to dissolve while I rushed into the kitchen to prepare some food for him when he came around. Had they been able to inject him, he would have regained consciousness suddenly, like a light being switched on. But because the glucose had to be administered orally, his regaining consciousness would take a bit longer. I quickly got a few sandwiches together and put a few biscuits on the plate as well. Paul was still unconscious when I returned to the lounge, but though the medics commented that it was taking longer than usual for him to come around, they didn't seem alarmed. Slowly, Paul began to move and looked up at all of us standing around him. He smiled, but was very weak and seemed a bit confused. Still, I knew this would all go away in the next few minutes.

Hoping for help

The ambulance men began explaining to Paul what had happened and telling him that he needed to eat some of the food that I had brought out. They then turned to me and explained that they had to stay with us until Paul's blood-sugar level was back up to six. Within half an hour, it was at five, so the ambulance men felt safe enough leaving and wrote out a letter for us to give to our GP detailing the incident. They told me to keep on checking his blood-sugar level throughout the day, in case it suddenly dropped again, but they didn't expect that it would. Earlier, they had given us the option of taking Paul to the hospital and of course he had refused that. As they left, Paul finished up the sandwiches I had made and told me that he was still hungry. That was a sign of low blood sugar, but I was happy that he was recovering so quickly. I went back into the kitchen to make him a cooked breakfast, starting with a cup of tea, which I took out to him in the lounge. When he was completely settled, I tried to get some more information about what had happened. He told me that he had forgotten to check his blood-sugar levels the previous night, which I found strangely irresponsible. Having had diabetes for so long, I didn't see how he could just forget one night to check his levels, but I didn't want to begin blaming him after what he had just been through.

Towards the end of October, I received another piece of mail from our friend at the hospital. This time it was the NHS staff magazine for the hospital. It was the current issue and in it was an article on the chief executive, who was being promoted to run three hospitals in another part of the country. He was quoted as saying how enormously privileged he had been to work with the staff at the hospital. "*The improvement that they have brought about in patient care during my time at the trust has been inspirational. I shall take what I have learnt through my experience here to my new environment and in so doing will be helping good practice in the NHS.*" There was also a quote from the hospital chairman saying that the chief executive "*has led the trust with enthusiasm and a strong commitment to ensuring that it provides the highest possible quality of care for its patients."* I know that people get promoted for many reasons, but still couldn't help feeling that this was the price the chief executive would pay for the way Paul had been treated - a nice promotion and removal from a bothersome situation. I wanted to rip the offending magazine to shreds, but I knew that it had been sent to me for a reason and maybe it would come in handy one day.

Ever since Paul had gone into hospital the first time, I had written a kind of diary detailing everything that had happened to us and since the negligence case began, I had kept all the papers encased in plastic wallets in rows of binders. I had many of them lying around the house now, hundreds of documents awaiting the day when they might be called upon to prove that someone was trying to deny responsibility for what they had done or cheat us in some other way. I had since learned that people were capable of all kinds of unfairness, even when they professed their best intents to you and seemed kind and caring. I hated being reduced to this paranoid state, but I would hate even more not to see justice done for Paul.

I received a couple of phone calls that day from staff at the hospital, asking me if I had found out that the chief executive was leaving. The general consensus seemed to be that he was being moved for his own protection. Perhaps the powers that be thought that if he was no longer at the hospital, then Paul and I would not be so keen to prove that we had been lied to about his 'missing' blood test results. They were about to be proven very wrong, because I had promised Paul that I would carry on fighting for him and all the other patients that were similarly being given poor care in hospital. Getting this copy of the hospital magazine reminded me of the last package I had received, with the mysterious memos about Paul's medical files being updated before the meeting at which the chief executive had claimed Paul had not been discharged in renal failure. I had been meaning to try to make some sense of them for the past month, but had been too busy dealing with Paul. I made a mental note to sit down with them and all my files as soon as I had a chance.

Hoping for help

Social services had finally made contact with us to say that a worker would come to see us the following week, over nine months after we had first contacted them. A week later, a social worker paid us a visit. After we had introduced ourselves, she sat down with Paul in the lounge. I went to make us tea and could hear her talking to Paul. I was glad that she was at least making some attempt to understand his communications. When I went back in with the tea, I asked her if she wanted me to tell her our story and she said that she did. So I began and finally got to the end, having cried at certain points and being prompted by Paul at others. She said that she had never heard of anything so horrific. I then told her that Paul didn't want to live anymore. As most people did, she looked straight at him then. He nodded and gave a very sad half-smile, looking down at his body by way of explanation. She had been making notes as I had been speaking, jotting down the particulars of Paul's case. She now put her pen down and looked at both of us and said, "this is my first case in this sort of situation, so I have to ask you to bear with me a little." Of course we both agreed, assuming that maybe she had worked as a social worker in a different field before. We explained to her the kind of care that Paul needed and asked about respite care. We told her that we were very worried about him, if something happened to me and I was unable to care for him. He needed somewhere he would feel safe and cared for. She said that Paul needed one-to-one care (as if I didn't already know that) and that she didn't know of any place with the type of facilities Paul needed, but that she would ask her colleagues when she got back to her office. We then asked her about some sort of courses for Paul, somewhere he could go to learn something new or do something so that he felt a useful part of the community again - maybe computer courses or something similar, anything to get him out of the house and feeling a bit more independent. She responded that she believed the main place local to us had since closed down and anyway she didn't think that any day centres would be willing to take on someone in Paul's condition, who needed such a high level of attention. Again, she would check with her colleagues.

Hoping for help

At the end of it all, we didn't really know what she was saying, as she didn't seem to have an answer to any of our questions. I got quite despondent as the meeting went on and she continued to tell us how unlikely it was that social services would be able to do anything to help us out of our situation. I got up to go to the bathroom and also to get Paul some saline as he was coughing badly and needed to go on his nebulizer. While I was in the bathroom, I heard Paul getting into his wheelchair and then he was at the door, telling me to hurry because the social worker was asking him all sorts of questions about him wanting to take his life. I made my way back to the lounge as quickly as I could, but by then the subject had changed. She apparently didn't want to discuss his suicide with me in the room, but Paul didn't want to discuss it without me there. I didn't want to force the issue though and brought up different ideas for caring for Paul.

"Well, obviously you will be able to buy the very best care for Paul once he gets his compensation, so that's probably the best way to deal with that," the social worker suggested as she closed her file.

"But his compensation might take years to sort out," I pointed out, "what are we supposed to do in the meantime? I have been taking care of him for years, with some help from my sons, but how long can I go on doing that? I need some help."

"I'm going to send you the addresses of some websites to look at," she said, "that way you can see the quality of care that can be bought. These are just for you to get an idea, as most of them are in Canada and America, but it should give you some information." She smiled at us then as though she was doing us a huge favour. I didn't see why she thought that we would want to know what Canadians or Americans do for their disabled, but I just thanked her and smiled back. I suppose I should have shouted at the top of my lungs that we needed help and we needed it now. I couldn't believe we had waited nine months for this visit, only to be told that Paul was too severely disabled for them to do anything to help. After I had shown her out, I went back into the lounge and Paul just gave me a look that said "don't even talk about it." Then he mouthed to me, "no one is ever going to help us." I walked away with tears in my eyes, saying, "let's wait and see what happens when she speaks to her colleagues." But we both already knew.

That evening I went to the gym as usual, while the boys stayed home with Paul. When I got home, Paul asked me if we could talk for a while. I can't say that I was looking forward to it, because I knew it couldn't be anything good, but there was no way I could say no. If he needed to get something off his chest, then I owed it to him to listen. He began by asking me about compensation money and how much I would get if he were still alive, versus what I would get if he were to die. I had already explained this to him in brief, but now he wanted all the details. I gave them to him as our lawyer had explained them to me. I summed it all up by saying, "in a nutshell, if you were to die now then you would be saving the NHS a lot of money. Many hundreds of thousands of pounds in fact." He seemed disappointed by this, but then asked, "but they will still have to give you a substantial amount of money if I die, won't they?" I didn't want to encourage him, but I had to tell him the truth. "Yes, it would probably be quite substantial. Depends on whether we settled out of court or not."

He went on to mouth, "if I don't make it until the compensation is settled, there are certain things we should discuss. Things that I want done after my death. To begin with, I would like Adam and Lee to be able to start their own businesses out of the compensation money. Probably not right away, but maybe when they are in their thirties and even forties and old enough to make the money work for them. It can sit in the bank until then. I would also like both of them to have lovely wedding receptions at my expense."

I could feel my face dropping. Sometimes I wondered if Paul was playing with my emotions, constantly talking about something so devastating as though it was a common occurrence. By now it seemed to be as frequent a topic as what we were going to have for dinner. How could he talk about it so often and still not have done it? Did he just want to hurt me? My head began to ache from all the thoughts swirling around in it, so I stood up and said, "we've talked enough for one evening."

"OK," he agreed, but I still have a lot of wishes to talk about. I would like you to write them down." I nodded. "Can we do it tomorrow?" he asked.

"We'll see," I replied and went off to make a cup of tea. That night, as we were getting ready to go to bed, I walked into our room to find Paul sitting on the edge of the bed, looking up at a very large framed picture of his father that we had on our wall. He looked up at me and I could see that he was crying. "I just want to be with them. Please help me." For a moment I couldn't move and then finally I broke down. I just couldn't cope anymore and went to sit with him on the edge of the bed, both of us crying and blowing our noses. When we had both calmed down a bit he said to me, "I mean it you know."

"I know you do, Paul" I mumbled tiredly. I really wished that this conversation would just end and that we would never have to have it again.

"I don't want to be here anymore. They will be waiting for me, both my mum and dad you know."

"Do you really believe that?" I wasn't trying to discourage him or put doubt in his mind, but I did wonder if he only believed that out of desperation. He had never been a very spiritual person, but I suppose the kinds of illnesses that he had survived change a person.

"Of course I do! Remember, I have died before," he mouthed with a smile.

"As if I could ever forget!" I replied, smiling as well.

"The only thing stopping me now is how to go about it so that it definitely works. The worst thing for me would be if I survived and had to go back to the ITU again." Then he turned to me and mouthed, "if you know I have done it and I'm still alive the next morning, could you put some pills down my throat to make sure?"

212

Hoping for help

When I could finally speak, I said, "Paul, don't ever say things like that. I want to be with you when you leave this world, so that you don't die alone, but please don't ask me to help kill you. I would like to do whatever I could to help you, but I am just not strong enough for that. I don't think I could live with myself, knowing I had done something like that, not to mention that I would probably get put in jail. Who would take care of the boys then?" I was starting to get a bit angry that he would even ask me such a thing and put me in that position. I tried to tell myself that he was just miserable and desperate, but I still couldn't quite believe he would do such a thing to me. "No, Paul, I couldn't. If you do this, you have to do it alone."

"It's alright, I wouldn't have wanted you to help, really. This is my choice. Anyway," he mouthed as he wiped away the last of his tears and then mine, "it's not going to be yet, we've still got lots more talking to do." I kissed him goodnight and we went to bed, but what had happened that night was still on our minds the next morning. We were both teary and silent all day long.

Paul wasn't too keen on going out around that time and had stopped keeping his doctors' appointments. He no longer saw any use for them. Since his health seemed to have stabilised, I didn't worry too much about it. I let the doctors know that he wouldn't be in to see them because he was depressed and they said that they would just reschedule for a few weeks' time in the hope that he would be feeling better about things then.

Later that week, I got a phone call from the social worker. She asked me if I had received the list of websites that she had sent for me to have a look through. I replied that I had and thanked her. I didn't bother to say that I couldn't see what possible use they would be to me. She then went on with what was obviously the main reason for her phone call. "I've just discovered a slight problem. I realised that Paul's GP's surgery is in Coventry and therefore his doctor would come under the West Midlands County Council. My area is Warwickshire County, so unfortunately I won't be able to carry on with your case."

Hoping for help

"But we live in Warwickshire," I objected, "so we are entitled to services from Warwickshire County."

"Yes, but since your doctor's surgery is in Coventry, there is nothing I can do but pass you over to their county council."

"So are you telling me that we will have to wait again, maybe another nine months, while someone from Coventry social services assigns someone to us?"

She began to apologise, but I just put the phone down. I couldn't believe that they would deny help to a person who needed it as much as Paul did on the basis of such a ridiculous technicality. And in nine months time, when they finally got around to assigning us someone from Coventry, I'm sure that person would take one look at Paul and then tell us they couldn't handle our case because we lived in Warwickshire. If Paul was even around by then to be looked at.

Paul had become even more removed now. He no longer tried to pick fights with us or hurl abuse our way. He had even given up on that. As I went about my daily routine, busy in the kitchen or bedroom, I would look over and see him sitting in his chair in the lounge, just staring at his hands folded in his lap. I would sometimes go over and put my hand on his shoulder and then he would look up at me and force a half-smile. When I left, he would go back to staring at his hands. I didn't even want to know what he was thinking about.

On Friday that week, our MP came to see us. He sat down to chat with Paul while I made us tea and, when I returned, I began showing him the documents I had received about Paul's "missing" blood test results, in particular those showing how on the 22nd March the chief executive had received a copy of the 27th September blood test results before meeting with us on the 29th March and claiming that the tests done on the 26th September were the most recent. I just handed them to him one by one, in chronological order and I didn't even need to say anything. When he was done, he looked at me and said, "if these documents are real, and they look to be, then this clearly implicates someone." We began discussing how to further the claim. We went on to talk about social services, but throughout the conversation the MP kept picking up the documents I had shown him and looking them over. I told him how our meeting with the social worker had gone and then about our subsequent phone call in which she had refused us any help. He thought I was joking at first when I said that her reason for rejecting us was that our doctor's surgery was outside her area. When he saw that I was serious, he became very cross. I also went on to tell him about the hospital prescribing the wrong sort of X-ray for Paul and he seemed astounded that the doctors were still making mistakes in Paul's treatment. As he got ready to go, he told me that he would be in touch with the chief executive of social services to try to get us some help and then would see if he could hurry along the negligence claim in any way. Then he looked at me and said, "what do we do about the new information about the missing blood tests?"

It bothered me to say this, but at the time I just didn't feel as if I could deal with any more than I already had to. "I would rather just leave it and concentrate on all the rest of the mess right now. We can't change that someone removed the results from Paul's file, but we can work on getting us a settlement and some help. Then we'll come back to this."

"It's quite near Christmas," the MP replied, "but I think this has to be dealt with now anyway. I think the only option we have is to go back to the police with the new evidence. Give me some time to think about it though, but I will probably contact them after the holidays, if not during."

I felt relieved that someone I trusted and who was in a position to help us, would be acting on our behalf and some of the weight was lifted off me. Paul and I wished him and his family a happy Christmas and then he left. Normally Paul would be a lot more optimistic after a visit from our MP, but this time he wasn't so convinced that he could help us.

Shortly after our MP's visit, our lawyer called to inform us that the NHS lawyers had offered a settlement of £150,000 "out of the blue". Although this may seem like a lot of money, it was nowhere near what we needed to get proper care for Paul – it was less than we needed to pay for Paul's care for one year. Our lawyer said that we shouldn't be discouraged. She believed that they had not yet grasped the full extent of Paul's injuries and reminded us that they always started off low anyway. As she put it, by this point in the 'game', patients were often so desperate to improve their lives that they would take anything that was given to them, just to get it over with and get some help. Paul and I found the whole idea of this being a 'game' for the hospital management, the NHS and the lawyers revolting, when we so urgently needed help. Our lawyer said that there was usually a bit of time between the initial offer and the final settlement, but it was definitely a step in the right direction that they had made an offer. Paul was devastated by their lack of concern and took it personally. "How dare they damage me this way and then insult me with such a low offer of compensation?"

I had no idea how to reassure him, because I knew that he was right. He felt worthless and inadequate, as he had done for most of the past two years. It's hard for me to put my finger on the exact moment, but if I had to pick one, I would say that for Paul, this was probably the point of no return. He no longer had any hope left.

Chapter 14

Waiting for the inevitable

Christmas was approaching, but for once no one in the house was really looking forward to it. Paul hadn't even mentioned it at all, when normally he would have been preparing two months ahead of time. We just went about our daily routines as usual. One evening I went to pick up Lee from work, leaving Paul home with Adam. When we got back, I got ready to go into the kitchen and start our dinner as I did every other night. When I passed the lounge, Paul looked at me with a pitiful expression on his face. "I want to go now," he mouthed.

"Where do you want to go?" I asked, thinking about the food in the oven and that it would burn if I didn't get to it soon. "We'll have to wait until after dinner, I have to serve the food before it burns." I looked at him, beginning to get a bit impatient when he didn't answer right away. Finally he said, "to die."

I didn't know what to say, so I just walked into the kitchen, crying. These days I was cooking all his favourite dinners, doing whatever I could think of to try and pull him out of his slump. Nothing worked and he spent most of his day looking at his hands folded in his lap or at the floor. I knew he was tortured and I was torn between wanting to help him out of it and knowing that there was nothing I could do about it. I didn't want him to suffer anymore, but there was simply no possible way I could help take his life. I began to get angry with him for putting me through this, thinking that if he were so miserable, why didn't he just do what he kept threatening to do, rather than dragging me through hell every day? I needed to be alive and well to take care of our two sons and if he kept on like this much longer, pushing me over the edge like

217

he seemed hell-bent on doing, then I was worried I wouldn't be around for them. I just wanted this all to be over.

We ate dinner in silence that night and then I got ready to go to the gym. To someone who has never been in this kind of situation, perhaps it seems cold of me to do so when my husband is in tears and wanting to take his own life. But he had been like that every day for months and months now and even if he didn't think his life could go anywhere, it did have to go on for the rest of us.

As the holidays approached, I asked the boys if they would mind looking after their father one Saturday while I did my Christmas shopping. Always willing to help out, they agreed immediately. So when the day arrived, I got together everything that they would need to take care of Paul – though by now they knew how to care for him almost as well as I did – and then set off. I called home to check in periodically and the boys kept insisting that Paul was fine. I phoned again on my way home, at around 9.00 pm and was told by Adam that everything was still fine and that his dad was going to bed. I found that a bit odd. "But he never goes to bed at this time," I pointed out.

"He's fine mum," Adam said, probably starting to get a bit annoyed with me being so overprotective.

"Well, I'm only twenty minutes away anyway."

"OK, but no rush. Really, dad's fine."

But I had a sick feeling in the pit of my stomach, even worse than the one I had every other day. I drove a bit faster than usual and got home at 9:25. The boys were upstairs playing games on their computer, so I yelled up at them to let them know that I was home. Adam came down the stairs. "Glad you're home," he said, "I've just been in to check on dad and he seems in a funny mood."

We both went into the bedroom and found Paul lying in the bed, fast asleep. I stayed with Paul for a minute, relieved that he seemed to be OK, but the worried feeling didn't go away. Something just didn't seem right, maybe it was his breathing. I'm not sure. I yelled up at Adam, "has Paul had his insulin and tablets?"

Waiting for the inevitable

He called back down, "yes, I gave him his insulin and I saw him take his medication before he went to bed." I opened Paul's bedside drawer, but the MST pills were still in there. He had one of those seven day medication organisers that I filled once a week and he had only taken up to Saturday. So that was all OK. Just as I was beginning to tell myself that I was being paranoid, Paul began to stir, but he wasn't waking up. A few moments went by and I realised that he was delirious. Immediately I thought, "this is it, he's finally done it." I thought about calling an ambulance, but I didn't. All of the conversations that we had had about his suicide came back to me and I could picture him pleading with me not to call the ambulance when he finally did it. He did not want to be saved. I just stood there for the time being, with my thoughts racing. There was no way I could have known beforehand how I would have reacted in this situation and I still didn't know what I would end up doing. Just then, Paul opened his eyes. He wasn't seeing anything though, he just lay there and groaned. It suddenly occurred to me that I had seen him look that way before and I ran into the lounge to get the blood meter. I pricked his finger and the seconds seemed like minutes while I waited for it to give me a reading. It was 1.9 – he was going into a diabetic coma again.

I had learnt my lesson from the last time this had happened, so I immediately put glucose tablets under his tongue and got a few of the bottles of glucose drinks that I had stocked up. Every time I could get his mouth open, I would squirt some in there. At the same time I had to pause every so often to wipe my tears and my nose. As the sugar began to take effect, Paul got very abusive. He mouthed some awful things to me while drifting in and out of consciousness and kept lashing out at me. I didn't stop trying to revive him though and I didn't call for Adam or Lee. I wanted to protect Paul's dignity as much as I could, as well as keep them from seeing their father in that sorry state. During that frenzied period, I didn't have much time to dwell on everything that he was saying to me and much of it was nonsense anyway. But when I thought about it later, it became clear to me that Paul had known what he was doing.

Waiting for the inevitable

I continued to feed him glucose until I got his blood sugar up to a normal level, checking it about every ten minutes until it stabilised. He finally calmed down at around 2.00 am and fell asleep. He said "goodbye" to me before he did, perhaps not realising that I had just saved him. For the rest of the night he slept soundly, not even waking when I pricked his finger to check his blood.

I was exhausted the next morning and left Paul in bed sleeping while I made myself a cup of tea. Adam and Lee got up to go to football practice and I cooked them breakfast before they left. I wanted to question Adam about Paul's insulin injection, but I was careful to do it in such a way that he wouldn't be suspicious. "Was there anything unusual about your dad's insulin injection last night?" I asked, doing my best to keep my voice casual.

"No, I just gave it to him as normal." There was a pause as he thought for a few moments. "There did some to be more in the syringe than normal though. It took a bit longer to squeeze in than it usually does. Why?"

Paul usually filled the syringe himself, especially when I wasn't around to do it for him. Adam wouldn't have known how much was supposed to be in there and even if he had, it probably would never have occurred to him to check. Who would think that their own father would try to trick them into killing him?

"Oh, no reason," I answered, "your dad just had a bad night, that's all."

After the boys had left, I sat in my chair waiting for Paul to wake up. I was absolutely furious. How could Paul have tried to use his own son to take his life? He had always said that this was something that he had to do on his own. What had he been thinking? I knew he was desperate, but I had no idea that he would sink to this level. What if he had died, how would Adam have been able to live with that? Paul had promised me that he wouldn't take his own life while he was left alone with the boys, but not only had he tried to do just that, he had even tried to make one of them responsible. I began to think that maybe I was going to have to help him out of this situation. Better me, than one of the boys.

Waiting for the inevitable

They were still so young. I didn't want either one of them to have to live with that. Just then I heard Paul's electric chair start up in the bedroom. I got up to have a word with him and as I neared the bedroom, I could hear him crying. Perhaps he finally realised how wrong he had been in trying to use Adam. As I entered our bedroom he looked at me and asked, "why?"

"Why what?"

"Why did you save me? I didn't want to wake up today. Why did you stop me?"

I went and sat on the bed next to him. "Listen Paul, I didn't know last night was the night. It's very difficult to leave someone to die. You just go into emergency mode and do what has to be done to save them. That's what I did. But what shocks me most about this is that you gave the injection to our son to give you the overdose."

He just looked at me, stunned, and then began sobbing all over again. "Oh God! I hadn't even realised. I was just so desperate!" He held his head in his hands and just cried and cried.

I was still angry with him, but I held him and tried to console him. It wasn't good for him to get so emotionally worked up, it might affect his breathing and then I would have to deal with that on top of everything else. When he had calmed down a bit, I said, "we have to talk." I made us both breakfast and afterwards, Paul drew up his insulin for me to inject. He began crying again and kept telling me how sorry he was about Adam. I didn't say anything, I just let him cry and smiled at him. I wanted us to talk without tears for a change, in a rational way, so that we could make decisions that we would stick with. I couldn't deal with this fear and uncertainty anymore.

After I got Paul showered and dressed and had taken care of his tracky and stump, I made us tea. I held his hand as he rode in his chair to the other end of the lounge so we could sit down for our talk. "I'm not going to mention about Adam again," I began, "because I know that you are suffering enough. I know you didn't realise the implications of what you were doing, but we can never let that happen again." He nodded, with his lip quivering. I continued, "Paul, I know you want to die and God knows I have tried to get help."

He interrupted me at that point with, "I don't want help, I want to die, that's all. I can't live anymore with all the insults and letdowns, the longer this goes on the more scared I get. It's never going to work out, they haven't left me any way out of this but to die. I know that's what they want me to do and maybe that's what's kept me from doing it for this long, but I just can't take it anymore."

It was hard for me to stay in control, but I knew I couldn't leave anything up to chance. "You have me," I said.

He began to mouth violently, he would have been shouting had he had a voice left. "You don't know how much that scares me, just the thought that I only have you to care for me. I know we have the boys, but I don't want to become a burden to them. I shouldn't have to rely on them. There is no way you can deal with all of this and care for me long term. What if you become ill? I don't want anyone else to look after me now anyway, no one else could do it without me being scared of choking to death. I can't trust anybody else. No one has shown any interest in helping to care for me and the solicitors and legal people are going to make this case go on for years. I can't sit and worry, scared to death about going into hospital and them not letting you care for me and then them leaving me on my own. No, no, no, please understand that I have to die, even the social services have left me to die and the doctors. Mandy, there is no way out. I'm certain that once I've gone, I'll be in a better place. I'm not at all worried about that. It's just getting it done that I am scared about. I'm so scared that I'll wake up and they will keep us apart and I'll not be able to attempt it again. Promise me that you'll never save me again."

"Why did you try to do it without my knowledge then?"

"Honestly, I didn't think I would be here today for us to argue about it. I can't allow you to be involved in this. You have to look after the boys and carry on this fight for me. Don't ever let this drop until you are completely satisfied with the answers you get. This is my life they have taken and it's not just medical negligence. They could have made up for that by doing the right thing, just once. But they didn't, they tried to hide it and wrap it up in lies."

"Paul," I insisted, "you have to tell me next time you're going to try to do it so I can make sure no one is involved and that the boys don't find you dead."

He stopped me there. "Every morning I cry when I wake up. We had a wonderful life, but that's been taken from us...."

I cut him off at that point. I had managed to remain lucid throughout our conversation and wanted to stay that way. Talking about the good times that would never be ours again, was sure to make me lose control. There were things we needed to discuss first. "Paul, can we try and get on with Christmas? Think of the boys – Christmas is always such a special time for us and if you die now, it will taint every Christmas from now on. Can you please try to stop these thoughts over the holidays?" I went into the kitchen at that point to start the Sunday dinner. It didn't seem as if I had managed to accomplish anything during that conversation. But a couple of minutes later I heard Paul's chair coming down the hall. "Let's go out tomorrow and get some presents for the boys," he mouthed. I smiled at him, "yes, let's."

The next morning we got up early and left for town. The mood lifted dramatically whenever we were out of the house. Like Paul, I was beginning to hate being in there for so many reasons. He had decided that he wanted to buy both Adam and Lee gold rings, so we started at a jewellery shop. We also picked out some clothes for them and, in a way, it almost seemed like Christmases past. Even talking about his death seemed a bit easier when we were out and he began now to get into specifics about his funeral. There was a song that was number one in the charts just then, called *Sorry* by Elton John and Blue. One of the main lines was *Sorry seems to be the hardest word.* It was on the radio all the time. Paul asked me if I would buy the CD after he died and play it at his funeral. I wasn't sure if I could go through with that, but I told him that I would see. I told him that I didn't even think they let you play your own music at funerals. He then went on to talk about his pallbearers and asked me to write up a list as we had lunch.

Paul bought us all extra gifts that year and, though we didn't have the money, there was no way I could bring myself to remind him of that. I was just glad to see him taking an interest in something again, even though I knew the reason behind it and it was devastating. He kept telling me not to buy him any presents as he wouldn't need anything. "Don't be ridiculous," I said, "how can we all sit there at Christmas opening our presents when there's nothing for you?"

"OK, but don't let the boys spend too much."

"I'm going to let them do as they like. Christmas is Christmas and if you are right and this is our last one together, then I want them to remember it having been as good as any other one."

In the week leading up to Christmas, Paul wanted to be out of the house as much as possible. I think he was worried that he would get so depressed that he wouldn't be able to hold out until after Christmas, as he had promised me. Often I would see him crying as he watched everyone else performing their holiday rituals, regretting all the ones he used to have that he could no longer indulge in. So we would drive around a lot or sit in the town centre watching all the people go by.

One particular evening, we sat on a bench next to the fountain in the middle of Nuneaton, listening to a brass band playing Christmas carols. The market was open late because of the season and as it got dark each stall had little lanterns hanging from the canvas roofs. I had wrapped Paul up very well and told him to just give me the word when he was ready to go home. We ended up sitting there for a couple of hours and it was a pleasure for me to see him enjoying Christmas again.

The band saw us sitting there and one of the members eventually came over to ask us if we had any requests. For some reason, that made me break down in tears, so the man just patted me on the shoulder and said, "OK, just carry on sitting there and listening." I wonder if he thought I was crazy. It doesn't really matter anyway, he was kind to us and that evening is a beautiful memory for me. It certainly helped me through the next few weeks.

Paul wanted to go over to the Coach and Horses on Christmas Eve for one last time. He asked Adam if he would mind taking him there and just pushing him to the bar. Of course Adam agreed, but then Paul backed out when the day actually arrived.

Paul had woken up that morning crying and was very pale. He would smile at the boys, but it was clearly forced. He wanted to go out for most of the day and I just couldn't say no to him. So I missed seeing most of the people who normally stop in for a quick bite and chat on Christmas Eve while out doing their last minute shopping. That included my parents. Luckily they stopped by later, after we had already returned home, so I got to chat with them for a bit.

That day, we drove around a bit more before finally going home. I think we managed to put on a brave face for Adam and Lee, but then you can never be quite sure. People often see much more than you give them credit for, especially when they are your own children. I had asked Paul to give his children one more Christmas with their father and I just hoped that I had done the right thing. I didn't want the day to be so horrible that it would taint the holiday for them for the rest of their lives.

On Christmas Day, I had set my alarm clock for 4.00 am so that I could get the turkey going in the oven. Once I had turned it on, I lay on the sofa in the lounge, mentally planning the day and thinking how I could make it happy for the boys. I made a decision that, for the first time in months, I would not cry that day. Today was going to be different, it was Christmas. At about 7.00 am, I began frying up bacon for my three men and found myself actually looking forward to the day. We had laid two crackers out on the table for Adam and Lee the night before, with a little surprise in each. When they opened them, Adam pulling his with Paul and Lee with me, the rings that Paul had bought for them fell out onto the table. It was lovely to see the looks on their faces when they saw their unexpected treasures.

Waiting for the inevitable

Breakfast went well, as did the present-opening and for once it almost felt like the way Christmas used to be for us. The boys had combined their money and bought Paul a lovely fleece jacket. It was a silvery-grey colour. After our breakfasts had settled, we all got up to get ready for the rest of the day. I had laid out Paul's clothes on the bed and as I was helping him to get ready, Adam came into our bedroom to ask us something. Seeing the clothes on the bed, he said "that's a lovely t-shirt you're going to wear dad." It was a new one, a beautiful beige material that I had hoped would put Paul in a more festive mood. After Adam had left, Paul turned to me and mouthed, "why not ask Adam if he wants that t-shirt."

"You're going to wear it," I said.

"Well, it's new and I'm not going to get much wear out of it, so let him have it."

I felt my stomach drop. Not today of all days. "Please Paul, let's not ruin the day by thinking about what's going to happen. We're all having such a lovely time so far and it's Christmas. Can we just not talk about it for one day?"

"I'm not going to talk about anything," he insisted, "I just want you to let Adam have that t-shirt to wear tonight."

I called Adam down. "Your dad said you can have that t-shirt you liked," I said, smiling at him and pointing to it.

A bright smile lit up his face and he quickly tried it on. "Thanks dad! Are you sure?" Paul nodded and Adam went off, pleased as punch.

"What are you going to wear then?" I asked Paul.

He wheeled himself round to his wardrobe, mouthing, "I'll find something." Out came his usual blue and grey sweat top, the one that he liked because it fit nicely around his tracky. I hadn't even thought that maybe the new beige one might not. "I'll feel more comfortable in this," he mouthed at me, smiling. I nodded. Suddenly he came around the bed and grabbed my hand. "Don't get rid of my clothes after I'm gone, OK?" I shook my head and walked away to the bathroom.

Waiting for the inevitable

As I was standing in front of the bathroom mirror putting on my make-up, I thought about how Paul had always been so fashion-conscious. He loved trendy clothes and always took very good care of what he had. If he went out anywhere, when he returned home he would never sit around the house in his good clothes. He would carefully hang them in the wardrobe for the next time he needed them. I wondered what I would do with all his clothes when he had gone. Some of them could go to the boys, if they wanted them, but what about the rest? I pushed the thoughts to the back of my mind, as I was trying my best to stick with my decision to have a tear-free day.

As I walked back into the bedroom, Paul mouthed to me "I'm sorry, I didn't mean to remind you. We are having a lovely day. Thank you."

I hugged him. "Yes, thank you too. We are having a lovely day. Now let's go to Vanessa's."

It was about 6:30 pm by the time we got to Vanessa's. In addition to the four of us, Abby, Lee's girlfriend, had joined us as well. Vanessa and Steve had done a lovely spread and afterwards we played cards and other games and sat around laughing and talking. Paul seemed almost like his old quirky self, which really pleased me. At a couple of points during the night Paul would say something that he knew was designed to stir up trouble between people and then he would look at me and give me one of his smiles that said, "got them arguing, now I'll back off and leave them to it." I would smile back at him, everyone knew him well enough to know it was all done in fun. As I looked around at everyone, I wondered if they had any idea of the mental state that Paul was usually in and how things were in our house every day except today. They all knew that he had wanted to kill himself, because I had told them, but did they realise how serious he was and how depressed? And how could the man who was sitting there, apparently having such a laugh, not think life was worth living? Again, I pushed the thoughts away. I would not give in to them today.

Waiting for the inevitable

As the evening drew to an end, Alfie, who was the boyfriend of my niece Leanne, asked us if we could give him a ride home. I explained that there were already the five of us in the car, but told him he was welcome to come with us if he could manage to squeeze into the back. We all went outside and as I was getting Paul's wheelchair into the boot, I could hear them all laughing in the back as they were trying to squeeze Alfie in. I went around to the driver's seat once I got the chair in and as I got into the car saw that Paul was laughing uncontrollably, as were all the kids in the back. I couldn't remember the last time I had seen a sight like that. Apparently someone had stepped in dog poo and brought it into the car with them. It stunk, but didn't bother Paul at all as he had lost much of his sense of smell and taste along with his voice. The rest of us weren't so lucky. Alfie decided that he would rather walk home than squeeze in amongst us with that stench, so he set off. The rest of us were trapped. The culprit turned out to be Adam and I called him every name I could think of on the way home and probably made up a few as well. Still, it was worth enduring the smell to see Paul laughing with the family again. I went to bed that night proud of us all for managing to enjoy our Christmas despite everything.

Boxing Day arrived and it was almost as though Christmas had never happened. Paul went right back to being his old gloomy self, staring at the floor and not speaking at all. I couldn't believe how abrupt the change was. As I was helping him get ready after he woke, he said to me "Christmas is over now." "I know," I said, walking out of our bedroom so I wouldn't have to continue the conversation. I didn't want the boys to see this reversal in their father's mood, so I was glad when they told us they would be going out that day. At least, half of the household could go ahead and enjoy the rest of the holidays. It was even worse now than it had been before Christmas, because though Paul had been depressed then, at least I had been reasonably sure he would do his best to wait until after the holiday. Now I knew that the time was fast approaching.

Waiting for the inevitable

We didn't go out anywhere between Christmas and New Year's Eve and as we got closer to the end of the year, I was beginning to realise that no one wanted to spend the evening with us. Perhaps I was just being paranoid, but as I called around to invite people over, they all already had other plans. Maybe it was just an unfortunate coincidence, but I couldn't help but feel that people were avoiding us and the black cloud that we brought with us. After all, who would want to start off a new year with such an unhappy reminder of the misfortunes that can befall someone with no warning at all.

We resigned ourselves to being alone at home on New Year's Eve. It was the first time – we always had people over in previous years. I wasn't sure I could deal with Paul on my own at such a time, but couldn't bring myself to ask Adam or Lee to stay home and "celebrate" with us. They got ready to go out partying and Paul gave each an extra £50 to help matters along. We settled in for a quiet night at home watching television, but around 8:30 Paul went into our bedroom and came back with a bottle of wine. He had got it from the back of our wardrobe, where we kept various bottles that had been given to us as gifts over the years. I never drank and Paul had stopped several years before, once he started on medication. But he came past me in his chair, clutching this bottle of wine in his hands and giving me a look that warned, "don't you say a word." Of course I did say a few words, along the lines of, "what are you doing? You know you can't drink on medication." "Who can't?" he replied angrily. "Mind your own business. I have to drink this to get through tonight and if it kills me, so what?"

We didn't even have a corkscrew in the house, so he just hacked away at it with a penknife, picking out the cork bit by bit. He eventually managed it, then sat there staring at the television until the bottle was empty. We didn't exchange any words the whole time he was drinking, but whenever our eyes happened to meet, I would flinch at the anger I saw in his. Later that evening, I got up to make some supper, thinking that if Paul had drunk an entire bottle of wine by himself, after not having had any alcohol in years, then he would need food to absorb it. When I came back from the kitchen with our plates of supper, he began to cry mouthing, "I've been a terrible husband, haven't I?"

I was really not in the mood to have this conversation – it seemed we had had it so many times already. I was exhausted and angry with him. This had to end. "No, Paul," I said tiredly, hoping my voice sounded more convincing than I felt, "you haven't been bad at all." We went back to the lounge and we ate our suppers in silence.

At the beginning of January, our MP rang me to ask me if I could go to the police station on the 11th. He had been asked to give a statement on the 'missing' blood test results. We were to meet with the detective at 11.00 that morning. Of course I agreed.

During those early days of January, Paul continued on much as before, staring at the floor or at the television. I don't think he was actually watching anything, he always seemed miles and miles away. We didn't talk much during those days and I just walked around with a sick feeling in the pit of my stomach all the time, waiting for the inevitable to happen. I tried to convince Paul to attend his various medical appointments, but he wouldn't budge. He told me that there was no point and he couldn't be bothered. He also began to clean out his paperwork and personal bedside drawers, tidying up and throwing out all the rubbish. I knew what all this meant, but what could I do?

On the morning of the 11th, I got ready to go to the police station. Paul wasn't interested in coming along. Although I had sworn never to do it again, I was forced to leave him at home with Adam and Lee.

When I got to the station, the detective showed me to a private room and we chatted for a bit while waiting for our MP to arrive. Once he did, he brought me up to date with what he had been trying to do for me and Paul, showing me letters he had written to various people who he thought might be able to help us. That done, we moved on to the new blood test evidence and the MP asked the detective what he thought of it all. The detective thought that it was shocking and assured us that he would investigate it thoroughly, but still doubted that he would be able to pin any criminal charges on anyone. I didn't do much talking during the meeting, as I could barely concentrate for worrying about what was going on back at our house. I kept praying that Paul would not pick this day to carry out his plan.

Once everything had been discussed, I asked the detective for some time alone with our MP. The detective left the room and I broke down, telling our MP that I believed that Paul was going to commit suicide any day now. I told him that there was nothing further I could do, since no one was willing to help us. He promised to do his best to get some assistance for us, but I think we both knew Paul was too far gone for that. The detective came back into the room a few minutes later and our MP told him that we were finished talking. I remember them both looking at me and I could see in their faces that they were angered at what Paul and I were being put through and embarrassed that they hadn't been able to do anything further to help us, despite their best efforts. "Is there anything else that we can do for you?" one of them asked me.

"What do I do when I find him dead?" I asked. They looked at one another and it seemed as if our MP was expecting the detective to answer the question. "Firstly," the detective began, "when a man says that he is going to commit suicide, then he usually will and there is nothing that you can do to stop him. Women can often be reasoned with, but not men. The standard procedure that you should follow is to call the uniformed police when you find his body."

Our MP interrupted at that point with, "do we really want that in this case?"

"It has to happen." The detective looked at me and I could see that he was racking his brains, trying to think of whatever he could do to make this the slightest bit easier for me. "Here is my personal mobile number," he said, "ring me if anything happens and I will try to be there." I wrote down the number with tears in my eyes.

Waiting for the inevitable

When I got home, Paul wasn't even interested in hearing how the meeting had gone, so instead I talked to the boys about it. Obviously I didn't tell them about the last bit, but I said that the two men were both going to make an extra effort to get us some help. They were relieved as they could both see that Paul was at the end of his tether. I wasn't sure how much I should be telling the boys. Was it right to encourage them to hope that Paul might pull through? Was it possible that he would? Even I didn't know at times.

Six days later I received in the post copies of the letters that the MP had sent out on our behalf. They were sent to our GP, social services, the secretary of state for health and the hospital. They were very strongly worded and I was touched that he was going out on a limb for us like that. It gave me hope again that there do exist officials and administrators who care about the people they are supposed to look after and are willing to work on their behalf. Even if it was too late for Paul, it wasn't due to the MP's lack of trying.

Vanessa and Steve often used to call at our house on Sundays, so I got up on Sunday the 19th January as usual, looking forward to a chat and a cup of tea with them. Paul and I were in the bathroom, where I was cleaning his tracky, but we weren't speaking. Relations those days were very strained between us – I never knew if I would wake up next to a dead body and I can only begin to guess at what Paul was feeling. As I was changing the dressing on the tube, Paul grabbed my hand and said, "I can't go on, I'm going to do it this week." I started to cry instantly, it was like switching on a tap. I had been living on the edge for so many months listening to him talking about his suicide but never knowing when or if it would happen. Tears were never far from my eyes, but I didn't know how many more of them my body could produce. I was simply sick and tired of crying.

"I can't take any more of this Paul. Please, just leave me alone. I don't want to know." I walked away and left him in the bathroom.

Waiting for the inevitable

He was very subdued all during the visit from Vanessa and Steve, not saying much and just looking down at the floor. At least he managed a smile for Vanessa as they left, when she leaned over and kissed him goodbye. I walked them to the door and when I had seen them out, stood between the first and second doors of our house, crying. I supposed Paul would just assume I was still talking to them. His words were playing over and over in my head. But they were the same words he had been saying for a year and a half. Was he serious?

I was never one to let matters go unresolved, so when I went back inside I sat down with him to try to explain what I was feeling. "I really can't cope with this anymore, Paul. The maybe of it all. Wondering every day whether I will wake up next to you and you'll be dead. Wondering how you will do it. I just need some time. I'm not running away from you and I will always be here for you, but can we please not talk about it for a while? I feel like I'm being pushed over the edge and if I go, then we'll really have problems. We've talked about it every day for the past eighteen months and I just can't take it anymore, OK?"

"OK, OK," he mouthed and that was all.

As I was preparing dinner, I replayed what I had said to him, not knowing whether or not I had done the right thing. I would never abandon him and I wished I could be there for him whenever he needed me, but if I wanted to keep my sanity, then I couldn't talk about his death anymore. Not right then anyway. I felt awful, but I just wasn't physically capable of doing it. Needless to say, things were tense between us for the remainder of that day. We had some more words at the end and Paul said something very cruel to me. "You just want me to do it, don't you? You just want me to kill myself!" I was so angry that I said, "Yes!" What's even worse is that at that point I think I meant it.

Maybe it was guilt, but the next morning I woke up with a renewed sense of life. It was a new day and I was going to do my best to make sure it was better than the last few had been. I would take Paul to the supermarket, where we could have lunch at the café there that we both liked. We would do our shopping, I would get him whatever treats he wanted and we would both enjoy being out of the house. I went into the kitchen to put on some tea and then back into the bedroom to wake Paul. I touched his arm gently, stroking it and said "Paul, please get up, we're going to go shopping today."

He opened his eyes. "No, I don't want to go."

"Well, why don't you get up anyway and we'll talk about it." I was hoping a cup of tea and some breakfast would make him feel a bit better. As we were eating, I said gently, doing my best not to seem as though I were forcing him, "we'll get ready and get going after breakfast."

Immediately he replied, "I'm not going. Don't you understand? I don't want to go to anywhere, I want to die."

I forced myself not to say anything and just gathered up the breakfast dishes. As I was washing up, I took deep breaths, trying to calm my nerves. I would try again. I just wanted to have a nice day for a change.

"Paul, please let's just get ready and go out. Let's try to be happy for a day. Please."

"No. You go on your own, I'll be fine."

"How can I go on my own and leave you here?"

"Easy. My breathing is OK right now and you won't be gone long. Go please, just go. We need shopping." He saw me debating it and pressed on. "Go on, go, you need to. I'll be OK. I promise I won't do anything while you're gone."

I gave him an annoyed look at that last statement, but I had to admit that the temptation to go out was strong. "I'll just go and get the things we need and then hurry home. But first I'm going to check and see what time Adam will be home. If it's soon, then I'll just wait for him."

I began to do a bit of tidying up and as I was vacuuming, I saw a posh car pull up outside our house. I didn't think anything of it, but a few moments later there was a knock on the door. I answered it and it was our GP.

"Have you locked your dog away?" he asked me first thing.

Waiting for the inevitable

I put Sheba in the bedroom and then came back into the lounge, where the doctor was smiling and chatting with Paul. I was hopeful that our GP would be able to do something to help us out, perhaps to get Paul out of his slump. But to my surprise, as I walked over to them, the doctor looked at me and said, "it's you I have come to see, really. I need some information on dates for your solicitor. Could you stop by the surgery later to run through some things with me?"

I saw Paul's face drop with disappointment and I hoped my emotions weren't as obvious. "OK, as long as Adam is home. I want to make sure Paul is looked after."

"I've also had a letter from your MP," he went on and I felt my hope rise again.

"Yes, I knew about that."

I could tell from his expression that our GP was upset that someone had talked to an MP concerning the care he was giving to one of his patients, particularly one that he had had for over twenty five years. But he turned to Paul and asked, "so how are you feeling?"

"Still the same. I'm depressed and I don't want to live."

"Well, let's see if we can give you another tablet that can make you feel better. They take a few weeks to work, but I'm sure they will help you. I don't have your file with me, because I came here to see your wife. I want to check to see if it will react with any of your other drugs first, so I won't give you a prescription now. How about if I go back to my surgery and check your file, then leave the prescription for Mandy when she comes to see me about those dates?"

I said "OK" and Paul just nodded. When the doctor had left, Paul looked at me and mouthed sarcastically, "a lot of good those letters are doing." I tried to be a bit optimistic, though I should have known better by then. "Well, he's going to give you another tablet and he seems pretty certain that it will make you feel better."

"If you go and fetch the prescription tomorrow, I'm not going to take them because they won't change my mind. No tablet can ever change the way this country has treated me and is still treating me."

There was nothing I could say to that.

As it turned out, Adam wouldn't be home until late that afternoon, so I decided I would run out to the supermarket to get the shopping. We worked out a system between us, where I would call every ten minutes. Paul would answer and tap once on the phone if he was OK and twice if he wasn't. Before I left, Paul asked me if I would get some minced beef to make him a shepherd's pie the next day with some baked cheese on top. I looked at him and smiled. It had been a long time since he had been interested enough to ask me to do anything or to show a preference. Of course I would.

All in all, I was gone about forty five minutes, but for some reason I wasn't panicking. I had already admitted to myself by then that, if Paul wanted to kill himself, there was nothing I could do to stop him. Every time I called, he tapped once and we even managed to have a conversation towards the end. I would ask him questions, but only ones that required a yes or no answer. Then he would tap accordingly.

When I got home, he seemed to be in a brighter mood. I thought it was because he had managed on his own for a bit and felt less dependent on me because of it. It led me to think that maybe I should begin leaving him on his own for short periods every day, just a few minutes at a time. Maybe tomorrow he would even want to go out.

The next day was Tuesday 21st January and I got up at 7:30 am as usual. I saw the boys off and then sat in the lounge watching television while waiting for Paul to get up. My mum usually stopped by on Tuesdays at around 10.00 am, which was just about when Paul used to wake up. Tuesday was also the day I refilled his medication pack for the week. At the height of all his illnesses, Paul was taking over twenty pills a day, but he had cut down substantially since then. Still, I would put the pills in his pack just in case he needed them. At the end of the week, there were usually quite a few pills left over, mainly painkillers and sleeping tablets. I thought I would wait until after my mum left and then refill it, as opposed to doing it while she was there as I normally did. This way, I would be able to chat a bit more with her.

My mum arrived and Paul came out of the bedroom to say hello, then just went and sat at the table, waiting for his breakfast to be made. He was obviously in a bit of a mood and mum sensed it, so she only stayed for about half an hour. I kissed her goodbye and walked back into the lounge, not looking forward to spending another day alone with Paul. As I got a closer look at his face, I would see that he didn't want to talk, so I thought I would just leave him alone until he was ready to.

I began to walk towards the bedroom, saying to him as I went, "I'll just get your medication drawer and we can do your tablets."

"I won't be needing them," he mouthed.

I was not in the mood for any more of his mind games, so I just walked into the bedroom and got the drawer. I heard him come up behind me, so I turned around. "I don't need my pack filled," he insisted.

"OK," I agreed, not wanting to start an argument. Perhaps Adam or Lee had done it last night while I was at the gym. Unlikely, but possible. Maybe Paul's mood would lighten a bit later and we could do it then. Or maybe he just still had a lot of pills in it. I would check later when he wasn't watching me.

I watched him draw up his insulin, checking to see that it was the proper dosage before injecting him. After the events of a couple months before, I had learned to be very cautious about that. I was relieved that he seemed to be carrying on his diabetes medication though, so at least he didn't intend to kill himself that way.

I made breakfast then and as we were eating it I asked, "would you like to go for a walk around town later?"

"I wish," he muttered.

He had chosen to take my words literally, which he almost never did. I thought I could take that response as a "no". "You know what I meant," I said to him, annoyed, "don't play." He didn't say anything, so I decided to just let him be. I was planning to prepare one of his favourite dinners that night, shepherd's pie, so maybe that would cheer him up later. In the meantime, I had lots of paperwork for his case that I needed to organise, so I would work on that instead.

By now I was continually writing to Tony Blair and various MPs, though none of it seemed to be doing us much good. They all liked talking about how important the NHS was, but didn't seem interested in doing anything to make sure people like us were treated properly by it. I kept and filed everything, so by now I had several large binders' worth. It was ironic that all of this had to do with Paul and yet he was not interested in any of what I was doing anymore. He wasn't interested in anything at all.

The rest of the morning went by without us speaking until lunchtime when he came to ask me to make his sandwiches. As I was doing so, he brought his chair to the doorway of the kitchen. He held something out to me and as I walked closer I could see it was his bank card. I had got him one when he received his first interim payment, thinking it would make him feel more in control of his money and his life if he could buy things without asking me first. It was a good idea, but unfortunately one that backfired. Because of his damaged left eye, he often couldn't see the numbers he was punching in and so would get his code wrong. His dyslexia probably didn't help him too much there either. Once he had got it wrong a couple of times, he would get flustered and nervous and then would hand the card to me to get the money out anyway. Now he was giving me the card back entirely it seemed.

"What are you giving this to me for? Do you want to buy something?" I tried to keep my tone light and hopeful, but I already knew what was coming.

"No. I can't use it anymore, can I? So you might as well have it."

"OK," I mumbled, taking the card and putting in on the kitchen counter. I was determined not to argue today and not to talk about his imminent suicide, if I could help it.

Waiting for the inevitable

After lunch he went to sit in front of the television in his armchair again, but he wasn't really watching. I continued with my paperwork, but would stop and stare at the back of his head every so often. I could see it move towards the window, then to the boys' school pictures on the wall, then down to the floor, over and over again. Some time passed and then he went to move into his wheelchair. This could sometimes be difficult for him to do on his own, so I went over to help him. He shoved me away roughly.

I knew what to do when he was in moods like this, which was mainly to stay out of his way, but to make sure I was always around in case he needed me. If he got too agitated, it might lead to breathing problems. And there was always the chance he would fall while he was trying so hard to prove that he didn't need help. I would try to be as innocuous as possible, pretending I was looking for something in whatever room he was in, but really I was keeping a close eye on him. But I wouldn't speak much, because that could really set him off.

I could hear him fussing about in the bedroom and then he was back at the dining table. In his hand was a pad which he had bought specifically for writing suicide notes.

"What are you doing?" I asked.

"Nothing, just some things I have to do."

"Who are you writing to?" I persisted.

"Would you just leave me alone and let me do this?" I could see that his anger was rising, but mine was too. I strongly disagreed with this writing of suicide notes, especially if they would only make the recipient feel even worse when he was gone. I knew that everyone was entitled to their own opinions and had a right to act on them, but I hated the thought of Adam and Lee receiving them and having to deal with that on top of losing their father.

"Look, this has to stop!" I begged, "you cannot write letters to our sons saying things that will make them sadder than they will already be. Please Paul."

"I just need to do this. I'll feel better when it's done."

Waiting for the inevitable

I left him then and went to sit in the armchair. I wondered whether he expected me to proof-read them when he was done. I was frustrated, but knew there was nothing I could do to stop him. He sat writing for about an hour, concentrating intensely. He wrote two letters, so I assumed there was one for each boy. It was about 4.00 pm by the time he was done.

"Do you have any envelopes?"

I went to fetch two and he carefully folded the sheets of paper he had been writing and put one into each. I asked him if he needed me to check them, but he said "no" and sealed the envelopes. I was worried about what he had written to our sons, assuming that's who the letters were for, but then I worried about everything these days, so it just slightly increased the sick feeling in my stomach.

I went into the bedroom then, because I didn't want to see what he did with the letters. I didn't want to know where he was putting them or anything else about them. When I came back into the lounge, he looked at me and smiled, mouthing, "I feel better now that I have done that." I simply nodded.

When I came back from the gym that night, Paul was watching television and his breathing sounded a bit stressed. He did seem a bit happier though and I liked to think it had something to do with my shepherd's pie. I hadn't had any myself as I have never eaten cheese, but he and the boys had really seemed to enjoy it. As I went into the lounge, he held out his hand to me. I took what he was giving me and looked down to see £70 in my hands. He would sometimes give me money to go out and buy him something, but not usually at night when it wasn't likely I would be going out again. "What's this for?"

"I don't need it."

"Well, neither do I."

"Fine, then just give it to Adam and Lee in the morning to get themselves something."

I put the money on the dining table and sat down to relax and watch some TV with him. It got near midnight and Paul began to get ready for bed. "My breathing is pretty loud tonight, maybe it would be better if you slept in the lounge," he suggested

"Alright," I agreed knowing that I would probably get more sleep that way.

I cleaned out his tube for him, then went to feed Sheba. I happened to walk past the bedroom as he was taking his pills and saw that he was crying. But I decided to finish taking care of the dog first and went to let her out in the back garden before going in to talk to Paul.

By the time I got back, he was lying on the bed on his side, so I sat in his wheelchair, rather than making him reposition himself on the bed. I held his hand and we sat talking until close to two in the morning. It seemed a very long time since we had done anything like that – I left the bedroom feeling closer to him than I had in quite a while. He talked about what he wanted me to do when he was gone. I hated hearing all of that, but I wanted him to say whatever he needed to. He wanted me to move out of the house, he said, which was filled with so many bad memories from the last couple of years. He wanted me to find someone else and get on with my life. I just said that we would see, not sure what I thought anymore, but wanting him to feel free to continue talking.

"One of the letters I wrote today is for you. Do you want to read it now?"

I couldn't speak for all the tears, but just shook my head violently, 'no'.

"OK," he mouthed and there was a long pause. "Would you give me a kiss?"

I leaned forward and gently pressed my lips to his. He seemed very relaxed, except for his nose, which kept itching. It made us laugh that he kept having to reach up to scratch it in the middle of our reminiscences. Somehow we had started talking about our past and what it was like when we first met and all the funny things that had happened to us in all the years that we had been married. As it got later, his eyes began to shut in between sentences. "You get yourself off to sleep now, Paul," I said, gently pulling my hand out of his and kissing him on the cheek. "Love ya."

I was relieved that a day that had started out so badly had ended up so well. I couldn't remember the last time we had just shared time like that. It was beautiful. I lay on the sofa in the lounge and cried myself to sleep, thinking of all the good things and all the bad things that we had shared. But I still felt a vague hope at the way the night had gone. Maybe tomorrow would be better and Paul would want to go out again. But I would never see Paul alive again. Later I realised that the itching on his nose had been caused by the overdose of MST that he had just taken.

Chapter 15

The hospital's problem is solved

Like everything else, I handled Paul's death and funeral in a very organised way. Never mind what I was feeling inside. The detective and a colleague arrived on the scene and relieved the uniformed police who had been called initially. He, in conjunction with the ambulance men, decided that our GP could pronounce Paul dead over the phone. How? I wondered. The detective was in the bedroom talking on the phone to our GP and from where I sat in the lounge, I could hear everything he said. He brought the phone out to me, judging it best that I speak to the doctor myself. I took the receiver and heard the gentle voice of our GP saying, "Mandy, I am so sorry."

"It's OK," I replied, not sure what else to say.

"Paul has died of a myocardial infraction," he informed me.

"Has he? How do you know that?"

"The ambulance men told me so."

"I don't think so," I asserted. I was not going to let them sweep Paul under the carpet like this. They had done it for the last few years of his life, but the real cause of his death would not go ignored as well.

"Do you want me to come over?"

Immediately I answered, "Yes!"

The detective and his colleague and I sat around waiting for our GP to arrive, while the ambulance men got ready to leave. Adam, Lee and Abby were upstairs and I wished I could be consoling my sons rather than dealing with all of this red tape. But I knew I couldn't take the chance that something would be

The hospital's problem is solved

overlooked. It seemed to me that they were already trying to deny that Paul's death was a suicide.

The undertakers came shortly after the ambulance left and went into our bedroom to prepare Paul to go to their offices. My mum and my brother Adrian arrived, looking shocked and concerned. I would have liked nothing better than to have mum hold me while I cried my eyes out, but I knew that I had to take care of other things first.

"I'm sorry mum," I said to her, "but Paul's body is still here and the police are waiting for the GP to arrive. Would you two mind coming back in a little while, because I really need to concentrate and deal with all of this right now. I don't think the police want too many people in here until this is all wrapped up."

They stood up and my mum hugged me, telling me that when she got home, she would call to see what was going on. I kissed her and she left. When the GP arrived, the detective let him in and the two of them went straight into our bedroom. They were in there talking for quite a while and then the detective came out to tell me that the doctor wanted a word with me. I walked over to where he was waiting for me in the hall.

He smiled, "Mandy, Paul has died of myocardial infraction."

"No, he has not. He's killed himself," I protested.

"Just let me sign the death certificate," the GP suggested, "it will be easier this way and then let them take Paul away."

I refused. "He hasn't died of a heart attack or myocardial infraction," I said again, walking back into the lounge. I tried to get the detective to help me and said to him, "Paul killed himself, it wasn't a myocardial infraction."

"OK, OK," he said, trying to calm me, "just sit down."

He went into the hall to talk to the GP and I heard the doctor leave a little while after. The detective then informed me that he would have to call the coroner. If Paul's death was suicide rather than from natural causes, this made the situation much more complicated for the police and the doctors. As the detective was on the phone with the coroner, I overheard him saying that Paul's

244

The hospital's problem is solved

body would be taken to our local hospital, the one that was responsible for all his problems. I immediately interrupted, "Paul's body can't go there, it will have to go to another hospital, any hospital, just not that one."

The detective then asked the coroner if it were possible to do as I had asked, but he informed me a few seconds later that it wasn't. Paul would have to go back to the local hospital. I began to cry for the first time since finding Paul's body. "How can we let him go back there now that he is dead? They were the ones who killed him!"

The detective reassured me that nothing further would happen to Paul. I suppose I should have known that he was right, as they had already done all the damage they could to him. He kept telling me that everything would be OK and since I had no choice in the matter, I had to believe him. He then informed the undertakers that they could leave, since the body would not be going with them right away, but to the hospital for an autopsy to establish if the cause of death was suicide. The men from the funeral directors had known Paul, one of them had even gone to school with him. Most of Paul's family had been buried by them as well, so they had known us for many years. The undertakers asked the detective if they could take Paul to the hospital, since the ambulance had already left and it would take time for another one to get there. The detective agreed and the men went back into the bedroom to get Paul ready. I was moved that they had offered to do this for Paul; so few of the people who should have helped us had ever done anything for us.

The kids came downstairs at about this point and were wandering around in a daze, careful not to go near the bedroom. After a few moments, the detective told them that they would be carrying Paul's body out soon and asked them if they would prefer to go back upstairs until it was done. They hurriedly agreed and vanished from the lounge. I just sat there watching the happenings as if it was TV. I wondered where Paul was at the moment. Had he stuck around to watch everything that was going on? Or had he rushed up to be with his mum and dad? The detective broke into

The hospital's problem is solved

my thoughts with, "Mandy, they are going to bring Paul out now, would you rather go upstairs?" I was a bit surprised that he would ask me that when, after all, I had found the body. "No, I'm staying here." The bedroom door opened and they wheeled out a trolley with a black plastic body bag on it. There was a zipper at the front of it that went from end to end and the bag vaguely had the shape of my husband. I followed them with my eyes until they went out of sight, then turned my eyes to the floor. Paul had left us.

I looked out the window moments later and watched as they loaded Paul into the hearse. Then the phone began to ring. I don't remember who arrived first, but suddenly the room was filled with people. My mum, Adrian, Vanessa and Nicola all arrived quite quickly. The boys and Abby came down from upstairs and my aunt Sandra and her daughter Melanie were there as well.

I asked my mum and Vanessa to help me change the sheets on the bed where Paul had just died. There were a few little blood marks on the mattress, from Paul's tracky and stump over time, so Vanessa suggested that we flip it as well. The police had taken the contents of Paul's medicine drawer with them, including the empty packets of MST and amatriptaline. I decided that I wanted everything out of the house that had to do with hospitals. So Vanessa and mum helped me go through the contents of the bathroom and get rid of all of Paul's medical things. It was then that I remembered we had a meeting that morning with the director of nursing and the man who was the hospital's acting chief executive while they waited for a permanent replacement for the chief executive who had recently been moved and promoted. The meeting was for 11.00 am, which hadn't come around yet.

I went into the living room and grabbed the phone. I got through to the director of nursing straight away and she answered in her normal chirpy voice, "hello Mandy."

"Hello," I said. "I'm afraid we won't be able to make the meeting this morning as Paul is dead." There was a long silence. "They are bringing him to the hospital; he should already be there in fact."

"Yes, OK," she whispered.

The hospital's problem is solved

"Could you please look after him this time?"

Less than an hour later, our lawyer rang. She seemed very shaken. She had just been phoned by the NHS lawyers. They had informed her that now Paul was dead, they were withdrawing their compensation offer. It had taken them months and months to make the initial offer, but before Paul's body was even cold, they had moved to take their offer back. At first I couldn't understand how they had even known about Paul's death and been able to act so quickly, until I remembered my phone conversation with the director of nursing. As soon as she had finished speaking to me, she must have phoned the NHS lawyers to tell them that their problem with Paul Steane and his family had been solved.